HOW FOOD
HEALS

HOW FOOD HEALS

EMMIE COHEN

NEW DEGREE PRESS

COPYRIGHT © 2021 EMMIE COHEN

HOW FOOD HEALS

ISBN   978-1-63676-358-3

ACKNOWLEDGEMENTS

Writing a book is something I never thought I would do. I had always appreciated literature, but writing was never my area of expertise. I am and always have been more enticed to the natural sciences. Writing lab reports was more up my alley, that is of course until I became so passionate about this topic. After I realized my chronic acne was derived from my gut microbiome and it was completely in my hands to fix it, I became obsessed with the idea that food can heal. If my acne, that I struggled with for seven years could be cured with the help of food, then what could this mean for people who struggle with more severe and detrimental health ailments. My curiosity led me onto the path of late night Pubmed searches, YouTube videos, and new recipes. My research started purely due to my curiosity. It wasn't until quarantine hit and I was presented with the opportunity to work with Brian Bies at New Degree Press and join Eric Koester's book writing fellowship that I decided to take my research a step further. My amazing and dedicated editors Megan Hennessey and Amanda Moskowitz helped me pursue this project, which was completely out of my comfort zone. When I realized that I had a story to share, research to explore, and a message to spread, I knew I had to write this book. I wish someone had given me a book like this seven years ago. Although I struggled with insecurities from my experiences with chronic acne, I am glad my story happened because if it hadn't, I would not be able to share this message with you.

I could not have done this alone.

To Jon Stahlman (MD), Darwin Deen (MD), Laurie Lewis (Certified Coach), Patricia Ischiropoulos (MD), Lauren Rosen (MD), Mitchell Cohen (MD), Karin Sargrad (MS), Kevin Skole (MD), Kim Joffe (MSN, CRNP, PMHNP), Myra Woodworth-Hobbs (PhD), and Elle Speed (LE), thank you for being such a critical part of my journey. I am extremely grateful for the insight I gained from our conversations and content reviews. This book would not have been possible without the expertise and knowledge you provided me. I will forever be appreciative of the time you have dedicated to me and this project.

I would like to thank everyone who generously supported me to make this book a reality:

Alana Agron, Anna Alworth, Emily Aronin, Gabbi Artillio, Kris Artillio, Barry family, Olivia Berger, Melissa Zietz-Berke, Leslie Berman, Joshua Boss, Boxman family, Shauna Brandman, Annie Brickel, Brzozowski family, Burak family, Woodley Burrow, Butler family, Cameron Campili, Camelia Carvajal, Missy Chapman, Lori Coffey, Rachel Cohen, Robin Cohen, Susan Cooper, Paul D'Amico, Daniel Deitch, Corina DelCampo, Abby DeYoung, DiCianno family, Mary Duffy, Katie Du Plessis, Marilyn Einheber, Ernst family, Jim and Dot Ettelson, John Everett, David Eyl, Ann Fandozzi, Felgoise family, Sue Friedman, Kevin Geisner, Rebecca Gerber, Anna Glowniak, Jan Gronemeyer, Judy Grune, Donna Harris, Liselotte Harrity, Carolyn

Hatoff, Debbie Heuckeroth, Joey Hodson, Gregory Horn, Lisa Kaplan, Kaufman family, Andrew Kelly, Ryan Kenneally, Paige Kokolakis, Karen Kramer, Jaydi Samuels Kuba, Alexis Lambert, Tierney Lanter, Jackie Lazzaro, David and Pam Lear, Ron and Suzanne Lear, Scott Lear, Lena Lerner, Brandon Lindsey, Powell Lowe, Lauren Mahoney, James Marek, Lecia Markowitz, Natalie Meltzer, Ilene Miller, Janelle Morrison, Alex Moskowitz, Ramona Naseri, Kathryn Noonan, Doug Olin, Jill Oster, Paladino family, Isabella Pantano, Brian Paul, Margie Paul, Josh Pardo, Barbara Pfeiffer, Debbie Poisson, Mindy Postal, Phyllis Pottash, Neil Ratna, Lindsey Reina, Melanie Reinhardt, Jackie Rogers, Kayte Rosan, Diane Rose, Rosen Family, Andi Samuels, Jonathan Savdie, Mason Schilling, Lisa Schlager, Kate Shields, Jordan Sternthal, Ben Swanson, Annette Swartz, Avery Topkis, Jamie Topkis, Logan Van Reken, Remi Weinstein, Jory Weiss, Werther family, Arielle Williamson, Vicki Wolf, Jonathan (MD) and Marsha Wolfe, Maxcine Wyman, Amy Yuter, and Cindy Zhang.

I am so lucky to be surrounded by a supportive family. Thank you to my uncles, aunts, and cousins: uncle Andy, aunt Diep, Jade, Dylan, Leah, uncle Mitchell, aunt Maileen, Jordan, Jamie, uncle Brett, uncle Todd, aunt Vicki, Rafe, Lexi, Daniel, Sophia, and Emma, and my loving grandparents Mom Mom (Zena), Pop Pop (Gil), Grandpop (Raymond), Zayde (Roger), Natasha, and Great Grandma Barbara.

Thank you to my incredible friends and family who took the time to read over my chapter(s) and provide feedback: Julie Klein, Frances Dovell, Christina Leonard, Ashleigh Acker, Dario Fucich, Michele Kaufman, Ryan Heaton, Tommy Weinstein, Jocy Spizman, Jordan Taxay, Talya Kalman, Vicki Pilgrim, Jade Bennett-Pham, and Dan SanGiovanni.

To Luke Brzozowski, my roommates Lindsey Grune and Sophie Tenenbaum, Steven Fandozzi, Bella Paladino, Adrien Gay-Bellile, Brandon Cohen, Julia Frangioni, Maddy Fair, and Natalie Paskin, thank you for continuing to support me when the book has been the only topic of conversation for months on end. I am so grateful to have friends like you.

To my dad, Barry, and my twin brother, Sam, thank you for believing in me and for trying all my new recipes. It is so easy to stay motivated and passionate about projects like this when I am constantly being surrounded by inspirational people like you.

Finally, a very special thank you to my mom, Sandy Cohen. You have been my rock throughout my journey, especially during the many days when I felt insecure. You always shared your positive outlook. You have always been real with me, guiding me down the right path throughout my life. This book would not have been possible without the many hours you spent listening to me and helping me put my thoughts on paper. You have inspired me to be the best version of myself and follow all of my passions. Thank you for your unconditional support. I love you.

CONTENTS

INTRODUCTION

———

Billions of dollars are poured into developing medicines to cure our ailments, allergies, and inflammations. However, sometimes these medications don't work right away or at all. Why does this happen? It's frustrating. What if it's not a drug alone that can heal us, but also what we eat? This is an interesting concept, right? Food is often thought of as a source of energy, but it can also be used as medicine for our physical and mental ailments.

I discovered the importance of food beyond simply being an energy source while I was struggling with moderate to severe acne. It took me seven years of obsessing over my skin to realize that the root cause of my acne was originating from within my gut and from the foods I was consuming. I had never previously taken the words "you are what you eat" verbatim. However, before simply describing my experience and helping others, I needed to pursue a more scholarly and research driven evaluation process of how nutrition impacts our gut health and our overall clinical well-being.

Ultimately, I want you to see this book as a tool to help you become more educated about the science of how our bodies both interact and intersect with the foods we eat. You should learn how to listen to your body to ensure you are eating a diet that aligns with your needs and goals. What I discovered has changed the entire way I see the future of health for our world: rather than starting with the entire list of healthy foods versus foods that raise insulin or increase fat, let's begin with the simplicity of the peanut. The peanut—and for that matter peanut allergies—has garnered global attention and forever changed the way lunches and snacks in elementary schools are provided.

In 2015, researchers from the United Kingdom and the United States (US) released a groundbreaking study on peanut allergies prevalence.[1] Having a peanut allergy is extremely detrimental to a child's overall health. A child with a peanut allergy must constantly be wary in order to avoid associated skin rashes, digestive problems, shortness of breath, and even anaphylactic reactions. Peanut allergies limit children more than you might imagine; they cause them to struggle with emotional, social, and spiritual health. It is hard enough for a child to avoid desserts but having to decline cake at a friend's birthday party, carry an EpiPen everywhere, and sit at isolated lunch tables takes a toll on their overall health. Parents became consumed critically assessing the ingredient list on food labels before purchasing and asking the servers at restaurants if peanut-free meals are available in order to avoid an emergency health situation. It is a formidable task to manage this issue in toddlers and to have your adolescent be mindful of the importance of paying attention to such details.

---

1   George Du Toit et al, "Randomized Trial of Peanut Consumption in Infants at Risk for Peanut Allergy," *The New England Journal of Medicine* 372, no. 9 (February 2015): 803–813; The National Peanut Board, "Managing Peanut Allergies," *Peanut Allergy Facts*, January 2015.

The prevalence of peanut allergies in 2008 was determined to be ten times higher among Jewish children in the United Kingdom (UK) compared to those in Israel.[2] This correlation likely points to an environmental cause to partially explain the geographical difference. Research later found that peanut protein was introduced, on average, at least four months earlier in Israeli children compared to English children: at seven months in Israel versus twelve months in the UK.[3] From 2000 to 2008, recommendations were made to pregnant women and new mothers to avoid peanuts when feeding their newborns.[4,5] During these eight years, rather than seeing a reduction in peanut allergy prevalence, US peanut allergy cases tripled![6] In 2008, the American Academy of Pediatrics reversed this recommendation.

The leading cause of death related to food-induced anaphylaxis in the US is peanut allergies. The American College of Asthma, Allergy, and Immunology in Seattle, Washington, reported that the US has one of the highest prevalences of peanut allergies in children around the world (2.2 percent or 1.25 million Americans).[7] To put this statistic in perspective, the number of children with peanut allergies in the US is

---

2   Ibid.

3   Ibid.

4   Ibid.

5   Trip Underwood, "Pregnancy and Peanuts," *Boston Children's Hospital*, December 24, 2013.

6   Scott H. Sicherer et al., "US Prevalence of Self-Reported Peanut, Tree Nut, and Sesame Allergy," *Journal of Allergy and Clinical Immunology* *125*, no. 6 (June 2010): 1322–26.

7   Tom Castles, "Pediatric Peanut Allergy Incidence and Prevalence on the Rise," *HCP Live*, November 17, 2018.

higher than the total number of children in Philadelphia. Other countries, such as the UK, have a high prevalence of peanut allergies, as well.[8] However, this is not the case for every country. Israel, for example, has a peanut allergy prevalence of 0.17 percent.[9] Why do we observe such a stark difference in the prevalence of peanut allergies between different countries?

An ongoing joke in Israel is that the first three words out of every toddler's mouth are *abba* (אַבָּא), which means dad; *ima* (אִמָא), which means mom; and *bamba* (בַּמבָּה), which is a popular peanut snack consumed regularly by children.[10] With an earlier introduction of peanuts into an infant's diet, peanut allergies decreased by 70 to 80 percent in the 2015 Learning Early about Peanut Allergy (LEAP) study.[11] Since common comorbidities in peanut allergy patients include eczema (63 percent) and an additional food allergy (35 percent), the study focused on infants between the ages of four to eleven months with either severe eczema, egg allergies,

---

8   Jonathan O'brien Hourihane et al., "The Impact of Government Advice to Pregnant Mothers Regarding Peanut Avoidance on the Prevalence of Peanut Allergy in United Kingdom Children at School Entry," *Journal of Allergy and Clinical Immunology* 119, no. 5 (May 2007): 1197–1202.

9   George Du Toit et al., "Early Consumption of Peanuts in Infancy Is Associated with a Low Prevalence of Peanut Allergy," *Journal of Allergy and Clinical Immunology* 122, no. 5 (November 2008): 984–91.

10 David Anderson and Rebecca Wilkin, "Why So Many Americans Are Allergic to Peanuts," *Business Insider*, October 7, 2020.

11 George Du Toit et al, "Randomized Trial of Peanut Consumption in Infants at Risk for Peanut Allergy," *The New England Journal of Medicine* 372, no. 9 (February 2015): 803–813; The National Peanut Board, "Managing Peanut Allergies," *Peanut Allergy Facts*, January 2015.

or both.[12] These specific conditions classify these infants as "high-risk" for peanut allergy.

Allergy organizations and the American Academy of Pediatrics (AAP) agreed on the new guidelines that emerged from the LEAP study, which included the recommendation of introducing peanut-containing foods early to prevent peanut allergies.[13] The FDA treatment option of Palforzia, used to treat peanut allergies, was approved in early 2020.[14] This drug may help reduce the risk of allergic reactions in children with peanut allergies. Currently, peanut allergies cannot be cured. Dr. Gideon Lack, MBBCH, MA, FRCPHC, a professor of pediatric allergy at King's College of London, discusses the prevention of peanut allergies: "It is much better to prevent the disease in the first place, and this is something we can now do for peanut allergies. . .much in the way we can vaccinate and prevent infectious diseases from occurring in children."[15]

National poor health outcomes and medical communication are suggesting that something is missing. The problem

---

12   Tom Castles, "Pediatric Peanut Allergy Incidence and Prevalence on the Rise," *HCP Live*, November 17, 2018; Susan L. Prescott et al., "A Global Survey of Changing Patterns of Food Allergy Burden in Children," *World Allergy Organization Journal* 6, (December 2013): 21. .

13   The National Peanut Board, "Managing Peanut Allergies," *Peanut Allergy Facts*, January 2015.

14   Office of the Commissioner, "FDA Approves First Drug for Treatment of Peanut Allergy for Children," *US Food and Drug Administration*, January 31, 2020.

15   *Craig Miller Production*, "Dr. Gideon Lack Discusses Prevention of Peanut Allergy," 2018, *Vimeo* video, 00:46.

is that we all think of food as fuel but don't realize that some foods have the power to heal as well.

Have you ever thought about or perseverated on a problem, over and over, for days, months, and years? You think of this problem so much that it even shows up in your dreams. Then, you suddenly have a revelation, and something triggers insight within you to understand or solve the problem. This is exactly what happened to me. I thought about the same problem every day for almost seven years. And the problem was my acne.

I developed acne—which itself was not uncommon—at the age of thirteen, earlier than most of my peers. I remember being very self-conscious and desperately wanting to hide my blemishes from the world. The only luck I had was with the Studio Fix MAC powder makeup, but it still could not fully disguise the amount of acne there was on my face. Unfortunately, my acne became more severe over time, and four, five, six years later, I was wishing I still had the acne I had when I was thirteen.

My family knew that I had sensitive skin the day I was born. I constantly had issues with my skin, from common heat rashes to eczema and rosacea. I started seeing a dermatologist at eleven years old to deal with my follicular and cutaneous predicaments and was prescribed countless ointments and topical corticosteroids to treat my dermatological nightmares.

I was constantly trying new medications, hoping one of them would be my savior. I tried oral antibiotics, topical antibiotics, gels, and acidic washes. Nothing worked! At fifteen, I was prescribed Accutane (F. Hoffmann-La Roche AG Basel Switzerland) for six months. The side effects I experienced included, but were not limited to, extremely dry skin, unrelenting nausea, loss of appetite, and signs of apathy/ depression. It was horrible but it also did not work. After using Accutane, I didn't know what to do.

It is common for everyone to have acne in some shape or form. I know many illnesses are more severe than "isolated teenage" acne, but this condition was negatively affecting my self-esteem. Compassionate friends and family were constantly telling me how beautiful I was, but all I saw and thought everyone else saw were the big, disgusting, pus-filled dots all over my face. I went on birth control, norgestimate-ethinyl estradiol, specifically to slow down the progression of pustules and pimples. I started wearing makeup on my face every day to school, despite knowing that even though the foundation may have eliminated the redness, it made the bumps more prominent and the inflammation worse.

Two years later, my skin had not changed. I still had moderate-severe acne. My friends had almost outgrown their acne phase, and, adding fuel to the fire, my twin brother's skin was perfect. The summer before entering college, I started seeing an esthetician, Elle Speed, for oxygen and HydraFacial therapy. Oxygen facial therapies are designed to promote collagen growth by spraying high concentrated oxygen molecules into your epidermis, the outermost layer of the skin. HydraFacial therapy uses patented technology and medical-grade devices to cleanse and clear dead skin cells, hydrate and loosen pores, and extract impurities from the skin using a mix of glycolic and salicylic acids. "HydraFacial delivers an instant glow. You can see and feel the results," according to Elle Speed. Elle was right, the treatments helped unclog my pores, but unfortunately, they did not eliminate my acne. I went to college thinking that my acne couldn't get any worse.

As a biology major on a pre-medical track at college in Atlanta, Georgia, I was immersed into a high-stress environment. Those factors, combined with the humidity of living in the South and the loss of home-cooked meals, caused my acne to worsen. At this point I was wishing I had the acne I had when I was seventeen. Everyone told me how beautiful I was and how they saw past my skin, but I couldn't. I lost confidence in myself and was constantly embarrassed.

During my sophomore year of college, despite my persistent and never-ending facial acne, I started to develop some confidence. I was passionate about my studies, I had amazing friends, and my relationship with my family was great. I regained the motivation and hope that I hadn't felt in years. I wanted to be healthier. My lifestyle became active. I worked out five to six days a week. I changed my eating habits. Thanks to a combination of a healthy lifestyle, a change in diet, and common acne medications (a round of doxycycline and Tretinoin cream, both of which I had tried before and failed), I was able to clear up my skin. For the first time in seven years, I had healthy, unblemished, clear skin. I remember looking at myself in the mirror, crying, a couple of months before my twentieth birthday. I never thought that day would come.

Although I don't doubt that leaving my teenage years in the rearview mirror helped facilitate such a change, I truly believe that my dietary changes and exercise routines contributed to this positive outcome. While the doxycycline antibiotic contributed to clearer skin, it was likely not the sole factor responsible for this newfound state of facial purity. When I took the medication five years earlier, my hormone levels were constantly changing and were now more balanced at the age of nineteen than they were at fifteen. However, I was on doxycycline months prior to changing my diet, and during those months my acne had not improved. Many acne treatments can worsen your skin at first, but this is generally not an issue with doxycycline.

I believe my lifestyle change regarding exercise was a major factor in clearing my skin because exercise produces endorphins, reducing stress. At the time of this journey, I was in a constant state of school-related stress. Stress-related hormones, such as corticotropin-releasing hormone (CRH), can drive up oil production in the skin, which causes acne. Additionally, small factors may have included the change in my location from the South to the North during the COVID-19 pandemic, the temperature change as seasons passed, and a reduction in makeup usage. There is no possible way to determine what single change caused my acne to clear up, but I believe it is a combination of the aforementioned shifts, with an emphasis on my change in diet.

During this time, I noticed the importance of food beyond an energy standpoint. I never felt like I had an unhealthy diet. Every person has unique "trigger" foods that cause their body additional stress. It took me a while to identify mine and to adjust my diet. In my case, most dairy, refined grains, and red meats caused my body to become inflamed. I believe the major factor in getting rid of my acne was cutting down on these foods and introducing a high-fiber diet to have a healthier gut microbiome. I went through years of medication and home remedies, yet the entire time, the issue was coming from within my gut! After identifying this relationship, I became curious about and invested in how food heals us and the importance of being mindful of the foods we eat.

Modern medicine will and should always be prescribed to treat specific conditions; however, it should not be the only medical option. It is incredibly important to normalize the idea that food can heal us. In each chapter of this book, I plan to help you understand the mindset of looking at food as medicine for our physical and mental health challenges. This book is written in three parts:

Part 1: How We Got Here introduces the history of nutrition and the "food can heal" mindset, explains the gut microbiome, and explores food-derived inflammation.

Part 2. Principles of the "Food Can Heal" Mindset contains chapters on gluten and grains, fats, dairy, and supplements. You will understand that everyone has an individual relationship with food and learn how certain foods can alter the gut microbiome, and therefore, affect your overall health.

Part 3: How to Optimize Your Eating Schedule covers breakfast and dessert to emphasize how the timing of your meals can have an impact on your health ailments and contribute to your overall well-being.

In this book, you will hear stories, such as:

- The fad of nut milks and whether they should even be considered as a milk alternative
- Scientific reasonings as to why following a gluten-free diet may not be beneficial to you if you are not gluten-intolerant
- How much truth lies behind common theories of breakfast being the most important meal of the day, and what actually happens in your body when you eat right before you go to sleep

Explaining the Scientific Reader:

This book is intended for all audiences, including scientific and non-scientific readers. I have created boxes to scientifically elaborate on certain points. Feel free to read these boxes to gain a deeper scientific understanding. Please note that you will still grasp the same overall message even if you skip these boxes. ☺

This book should not be interpreted as medical advice. Please consult with your health care providers regarding any medical issues and changes to your diet.

ONE

HOW WE
GOT HERE

ONE

THE RISE OF NUTRITION

———

"Let food be thy medicine and medicine be thy food."

- HIPPOCRATES (400 BCE)[16]

We cannot master the practice of the food can heal mindset overnight; much more effort is required to adopt this lifestyle. Science has singlehandedly emphasized the importance of the food can heal mindset, and yet, we consistently ignore it despite its proven benefits to quality of life and health.

Interestingly, the concept of how food can heal dates back to Hippocrates, the father of medicine. Hippocrates was the first to investigate how diet influences health, since he believed all illnesses arose from natural causes. If only science-based evidence existed supporting the relationship of food and human health back in the fifth century BCE, maybe we would live in a world where everyone was taught and understood the importance of nutrition.

———

16   Mark Lucock, "Is Folic Acid the Ultimate Functional Food Component for Disease Prevention?," *BMJ 328*, no. 7422 (2004): 211–4.

How can science-based evidence about something as important as the idea that food can heal still not be widely accepted today? To understand the current state of nutrition, I want to go back in time and explain how we got here.

Today, doctors are honored and highly regarded. However, this was not always the case. Doctors used to be feared and distrusted. During the Medieval period (fifth to fifteenth century), most people never saw doctors. Treating ailments and disease revolved around magic and witchcraft. In medical school, doctors studied history and ancient Greek medicine. Simple leg infections were treated by amputation.[17] Bloodletting, which uses leeches to bleed the patient, was also a common treatment for many ailments. Patients went to barbers to get their teeth pulled, and the only medicines thought to cure disease were herbs. Religion was thought to help the mentally ill drive away evil spirits, and medicine was centered around spirituality.[18]

In 1747, one of the most dangerous adventures was the long sea voyage.[19] The greatest threat on these voyages wasn't the unpredictable weather, the violent pirates, nor the wars; it was something much more detrimental—food. During this period, sailors knew the risk of being exposed to scurvy, a disease caused by a lack of vitamin C. The death rate from scurvy on these voyages was 50 percent.[20] When historian

---

17 MNT Editorial Team, "What was Medieval and Renaissance Medicine?," *Medical News Today*, November 2, 2018.

18 "The Knight With the Lion: What Kind of Medicine Did People Use in the Middle Ages?," *University of Aberdeen*, accessed February 17, 2021.

19 "The History of Nutrition," *Natural Healers (Blog)*, accessed February 17, 2021.

20 Catherine Price, "The Age of Scurvy," *Science History Institute*, August 14, 2017.

Stephen Bown describes the search for a cure for scurvy, he describes it to be "a vital factor determining the destiny of nations."[21] Bown reports a survival story from an unknown surgeon during a sixteenth century English voyage: "It rotted all my gums, which gave out a black and putrid blood. . .I was forced to use my knife each day to cut into the flesh in order to release the black and foul blood of my lower legs. . . We saw bodies thrown into the sea constantly, three or four at a time."[22]

James Lind was the first to research scurvy's causes by experimenting with food.[23] He observed that the people dying of the disease were only eating nonperishables (e.g., bread and canned foods). He identified that individuals who ate citrus fruits were the only ones to recover from scurvy. Although Lind could not articulate his findings (since vitamin C was not discovered until nearly two centuries after his work), his ideas forever changed the importance of food as it uncovered a connection with food as medicine. In addition, many other early researchers linked nutrition to human health with the discovery of vitamin deficiencies such as beriberi (a lack of vitamin B1, Thiamin) and rickets (a lack of vitamin D).

For the Scientific Reader:
Scientific and medical development through the Enlightenment and Victorian age continually

---

21 "The History of Nutrition," *Natural Healers (Blog)*, accessed February 17, 2021.

22 Ibid.

23 "The Knight With the Lion: What Kind of Medicine Did People Use in the Middle Ages?," *University of Aberdeen*, accessed February 17, 2021.

introduced the healing powers of food. Antoine Lavoisier, the "father of nutrition and chemistry," created the concept of metabolism, the creation of energy through the transfer of food and oxygen into heat and water in the body.[24] Around this time, the main elements of food included carbon, nitrogen, hydrogen, and oxygen.[25] Researchers started investigating the chemical nature of carbohydrates, fats, proteins, and vitamins to explain food's effects on the body through its biological and chemical interactions.

We have come a long way since the Medieval era of medical practices. Identifying foods' impact on common vitamin deficiency diseases sparked interest in learning more about how food can heal.

THE NUTRITION LABEL

Today, many individuals are unaware of the foods they are putting into their bodies and how they affect their health. However, if they are interested in learning, they can start by looking at the nutrition label on food packaging. Nutrition labels should not be taken for granted. We are lucky to have them at our disposal, as this was not always the case. Food labels were not needed when the products were made of pure ingredients, including wheat, water, or salt.[26] However, as ingredients like monosodium glutamate were introduced,

---

24 Ibid.

25 Ibid.

26 Institute of Medicine, *Front-of-Package Nutrition Rating Systems and Symbols: Phase I Report* (Washington DC: National Academies Press, 2010).

consumers began to request additional information about what they were eating.[27]

Food manufacturers were eager to respond to the public's desires—although, perhaps a little bit too eager . . .

Manufacturing companies created undefined claims to catch the attention of their consumers.[28] Statements such as "extremely low in saturated fat" arose without a true understanding of what that really meant.[29] In 1984, Kellogg partnered with the National Cancer Institute to challenge the old policies and promote the benefits of a low fat, high fiber diet. Kellogg was the first cereal company to voluntarily share their products' sugar content on the side panel of their packaging.[30] The demand for high-fiber cereals reached new heights during these times. In response, around two million more households consumed high fiber cereals.

In 1990, the Food and Drug Administration (FDA) approved the Nutrition Labeling and Education Act (NLEA), which required foods to provide nutritional information with consistent claims.[31] With these new guidelines, a foundation for uniform nutrition labels became established. Nutrition labels must follow specific standards for health claims, so

---

27 Ibid.

28 Christine Lewis Taylor and Virginia L. Wilkening, "How the Nutrition Food Label Was Developed, Part 1," *Journal of the American Dietetic Association* 108, no. 3 (March 2008): 437–42.

29 Ibid.

30 "From Feeding the US Army to Going to the Moon to Making Everyday Moments G-r-r-r-Eat!," *Kellogg*, accessed February 17, 2021.

31 Henry A. Waxman, "H.R.3562 - 101st Congress (1989–1990): Nutrition Labeling and Education Act of 1990," *Congress.gov*, November 8, 1990.

companies could not arbitrarily dictate, for example, what "high fiber" meant. Additional requirements included reporting the serving size, total kilocalories, total fat (specifically, saturated and trans fats), sodium, sugars, total carbohydrates, cholesterol, dietary fiber, iron, calcium, and vitamins (e.g., A and C). The NLEA has been updated and revised since 1990, incorporating the following changes: uniform serving size, percent daily value, uniform definitions for descriptive labels, such as "light" and "fat-free," and the presence of eight common allergens (milk, eggs, fish, shellfish, tree nuts, peanuts, wheat, and soybeans).[32]

As you can see, establishing nutritional standards was not an easy process. Just as nutritional science took time to develop, so did the proper nutrition label. Here's an overview of the timeline:[33]

- 1906: The Pure Food and Drug Act led to the creation of the FDA and helped ban mislabeled products.

---

32   Institute of Medicine, *Front-of-Package Nutrition Rating Systems and Symbols: Phase I Report* (Washington DC: National Academies Press, 2010).

33   Sandy Skrovan, "The Origins and Evolution of Nutrition Facts Labeling," *Food Dive*, October 16, 2017; Institute of Medicine, *Front-of-Package Nutrition Rating Systems and Symbols: Phase I Report* (Washington DC: National Academies Press, 2010); Alyssa Pike et al., "The Nutrition Facts Label: Its History, Purpose and Updates," *Food Insight*, March 9, 2020; National Archives, "White House Conference on Food, Nutrition and Health (White House Central Files: Staff Member and Office Files)," White House Conference on Food, Nutrition and Health, *Richard Nixon Presidential Library and Museum*, accessed February 17, 2021.

- 1938: The Food, Drug, and Cosmetic Act required the reporting of all chemical preservatives, including artificial flavorings, and promoted the importance of a scientifically backed nutrition claim.
- 1969: The White House Conference on Food, Nutrition, and Health recommended that the FDA develop a system to help consumers identify the nutritional standard and characteristics of food.
- 1973: The FDA published their first nutrition label regulations.
- 1990: The Nutrition Labeling and Education Act proposed uniform regulations for a mandated nutrition label to follow.
- 1994: The Nutrition Facts panel (the nutrition label we see today) appeared on all food items in the US.

Nutrition labeling is a great tool for individuals to use to learn about what they are eating. Learning how to appropriately use a nutrition label will help you choose the food items that are most suitable for your healthy diet.

PREDICTIVE MEDICINE

How can we further incorporate the power of nutrition? The answer may be to integrate it with predictive medicine.

Over ten years ago, the idea of predictive medicine was highly speculated. The thought that positive health outcomes could be predicted was only hypothetical; the reality was reactive disease treatment.[34] It was not until 2003 when sci-

---

34   Mauricio Flores et al., "P4 Medicine: How Systems Medicine Will Transform the Healthcare Sector and Society," *Personalized Medicine* 10, no. 6 (August 2013): 565–76.

entists were able to complete a genetic blueprint of humans through the human genome project that people saw its potential.[35] Today, we are living in a time where predictive medicine is on the rise. With all the historical data available on past diseases, we can analyze and use this information to create personalized health plans for individuals. It is a fairly simple thought that people would live a healthier life if they did not get ill. While certain factors like genetics, which are associated with aging and disease, are uncontrollable, others are not.

If only there was a way to control the risk factors of diseases, such as hypertension (high blood pressure), hyper-cholesterolemia (high cholesterol), obesity, blood glucose levels, dyslipidemia (abnormal amount of lipids/fats), and more.

Oh, wait. . . there is.

The answer brings us back to Hippocrates' original thought: **Food can heal us.**

Your diet affects your overall health and may be used to proactively prevent diseases. Science has proven this. Unfortunately, a blind spot exists; people are not utilizing the food can heal mindset when choosing the foods they eat. Nutrition is not fully incorporated into modern education and practice. Relating to my personal experience with chronic acne, after years of failed medications, why was my diet not a main point of conversation at my doctor's appointments? Why isn't diet on a checklist of questions to ask all patients before discussing their health issues?

---

35   "The Human Genome Project." *NIH: National Human Genome Research Institute*, accessed February 17, 2021.

"To eat is a necessity, but to eat
intelligently is an art."[36]

- LA ROCHEFOUCAULD

I hope to live to a day when everyone is taught the importance of food and how we can use food to heal. A day when doctors in any field will ask about diet as part of your medical history. The importance of a patient's diet is just as important as recording past surgeries, smoking history, and quantity of alcohol consumption. At each future doctor's visit, I plan to discuss my diet, and I hope that you do, too. This action may help influence our doctors to include it in their conversations with all of their patients.

---

36   "The History of Nutrition," *Natural Healers (Blog)*, accessed February 17, 2021.

TWO

GUT MICROBIOME

———

*"Future strategies to target and treat chronic
diseases, including brain health, may depend
on targeting or feeding our gut microbiomes."*[37]

We are all familiar with that sensation of having a gut feeling,
that difficult-to-describe intuitive feeling. I always had a gut
feeling that I was overlooking something to improve my acne
and was surprised when I realized it actually involved my
gut. After researching more on this topic, I found myself
able to influence my gut health and, subsequently, clear my
acne. I learned that many of our health issues are directly
correlated to the health of our gut, more specifically, our gut
microbiome. Our gut microbiome and the foods we eat play
an important role in maintaining a healthy body. Here's why.

There are thirty trillion human cells in your body. This
may seem like a lot until you learn that there are thirty-eight

———

37   *TED*, "Ruairi Robertson: Food for Thought: How Your Belly Controls
      Your Brain," December 7, 2015, video, 14:30.

trillion *bacterial* cells in your body.[38] If you have ever heard the saying, "you are more bacteria than human," that's why. Since bacteria make up a large composition of the human body, it makes sense that their health is critical for our overall well-being. Bacteria are classified as a microorganism, along with viruses, fungi, and other microscopic livings. The different microorganisms present together in a specific environment are referred to as the microbiota. For example, all of the microorganisms found in the intestines would be referred to as the gut microbiota. The microbiome consists of all of the microorganisms in and on our body and their genetic material; this can be separated based on location. If we were to weigh the human microbiome, it would be around one to two kilograms (two to five pounds). This is around the same weight as your brain. The bulk of these microorganisms and their genes are condensed in the cecum, which is the space between the large and small intestines. This is your gut microbiome.

"Think of your gut microbiome as a second brain."

- DR. RUAIRI ROBERTSON, A LEADING RESEARCHER OF THE GUT MICROBIOME AT QUEEN MARY UNIVERSITY OF LONDON[39]

---

38   Rob Sender et al., "Revised Estimates for the Number of Human and Bacteria Cells in the Body," *PLoS Biology 14*, no. 8 (August 2016): e1002533.

39   *TED*, "Ruairi Robertson: Food for Thought: How Your Belly Controls Your Brain," December 7, 2015, video, 14:30.

Physically, the vagus nerve is able to send messages between the gut (the organs that make up the digestive tract) and the brain.[40] Biochemically, the two are similarly connected, with their relationship being extremely complex. Have you ever been really nervous and experienced "butterflies in your stomach"? Have you ever wondered what is going on? Can the stomach really synthesize feelings and emotions? Dr. Robertson believes that learning more about this relationship and having a general understanding of the gut microbiome are key to living a healthy life.

Despite the brain having billions of neurons that tell the body how to function and behave, the gut microbiome is believed to have a "mind of its own."[41] It can be argued that the gut microbiome can determine our actions and moods even more than our brains do. On a similar note, we also have more power to control our gut microbiome than we do to control our brain. In fact, 90 percent of the serotonin levels in your body are actually produced in the intestines.[42]

For the Scientific Reader:

This is why serotonin reuptake inhibitors (SSRIs) and serotonin-norepinephrine reuptake inhibitors (SNRIs), two different antidepressant medications, are commonly associated with gastrointestinal (GI) side effects. Both SSRIs and SNRIs are affected by

---

40   Ruairi Robertson, "The Gut-Brain Connection: How It Works and the Role of Nutrition," *Healthline*, last modified August 20, 2020.

41   *TED*, "Ruairi Robertson: Food for Thought: How Your Belly Controls Your Brain," December 7, 2015, video, 14:30.

42   Jessica Stoller-Conrad, "Microbes Help Produce Serotonin in Gut," *California Institute of Technology*, April 9, 2015.

serotonin levels. Since serotonin plays an important role in the motility of the GI tract, where a large prevalence of the serotonin in our body is found, drugs such as SSRI and SNRI, which influence serotonin receptors, can cause GI discomfort. [43]

This means that less than 10 percent of serotonin levels are actually coming from our brain. Since serotonin is associated with mood stability, low levels can be indicative of depression. The gut microbiome contains millions of neurons, and it is the center of the immune system.[44] If your gut microbiome is disturbed, this can trigger immune reactions throughout the body, including the brain. The longer the gut microbiome is disturbed, the greater the potential for negative effects to your health.[45]

It is essential to have a healthy relationship with the microorganisms inside your gut microbiome in an effort to coexist and mutually benefit. Trillions of microorganisms

---

43   Michael D. Gershon, "5-Hydroxyttryptamine (Serotonin) in the Gastrointestinal Tract," *Current Opinion in Endocrinology 20*, no. 1 (February 2013): 14–21; P Janssen et al., "The Influence of Citalopram on Interdigestive Gastrointestinal Motility in Man," *Alimentary Pharmacology and Therapeutics 32*, no. 2 (June 2010): 289–295; James M. Ferguson, "SSRI Antidepressant Medications: Adverse Effects and Tolerability," *Primary Care Companion to the Journal of Clinical Psychiatry 3*, no. 1 (February 2001) 22–27; Daniel Santarsieri and Thomas L Schwartz, "Antidepressant Efficacy and Side-Effect Burden: A Quick Guide for Clinicians," *Drugs in Context 4*, (October 2015): 212290.

44   Helen Fields, "The Gut: Where Bacteria and Immune System Meet," *John Hopkins Medicine*, November 2015.

45   Ibid.

are surviving off your body and the food that you eat. As an interconnected ecosystem, the food we eat and bring into our digestive system feeds the microbes living in our gut. Reciprocally, these microbes produce nutrients, such as vitamin K, which are essential for healthy development and well-being. This knowledge is not new; however, it is believed that back in the late nineteenth and early twentieth centuries, a man by the name of Ilya Mechnikov may have been the first to learn of our internal ecosystem.[46] Unfortunately for Mechnikov, his ideas were not well-received in his lifetime. However, he is now considered a hero by me and by people all over the world.[47] In the nutritional world, it is very common for scientifically proven ideas to take a while to normalize. I will mention a lot of these ideas in the book. My goal is that the concept of using food to heal will assimilate into society within a shorter period of time than some of the previous ideas which, in some cases, took as long as three centuries.

The appropriate balance of microorganisms in our gut microbiome may be a major factor in helping fight off diseases.[48] Mechnikov recognized inflammation's ability to act as a biological self-defense mechanism. However, this idea was very foreign.[49] Inflammation had only been associated with diseases. At this time, the humoral theory dominated.[50]

---

46 Ibid.

47 *TED*, "Ruairi Robertson: Food for Thought: How Your Belly Controls Your Brain," December 7, 2015, video, 14:30.

48 Ibid.

49 Valerie Racine, "Ilya Ilyich Mechnikov (Elie Metchnikoff) (1845–1916)," *The Embryo Project Encyclopedia*, July 5, 2014.

50 Ibid; "Ilya Mechnikov: Nobel Lecture," *The Nobel Prize*, December 11, 1908.

The term "humoral" relates to "humors," which is a way of looking at the body from the time after Hippocrates. Contrary to the ideas of Mechnikov, the humoral theory stated that phagocytes (cells with digestive functions) were harmful, as they were blamed as the culprit of spreading diseases.[51] Mechnikov's theory believed phagocytes provided defense mechanisms against foreign invasions to the body.[52] Mechnikov's discoveries struggled to receive the recognition they deserved because they opposed the society of that time's beliefs.

The immune system is highly complex, which explains why it took so long to understand it and to make its connection to our gut health, specifically, the gut microbiome. The microorganisms that occupy our gut microbiome have thousands of different functions.[53] They digest foods, produce vitamins and hormones, provide key responses to drugs and infections, and help control blood cholesterol and sugar levels.[54] With 70 to 80 percent of the immune system inhabiting our gut microorganisms, how can we ensure we are working together with our gut microbiome?[55] Chronic inflammation and diseases often stem from a toxic relationship with our gut microbiome.

51   Valerie Racine, "Ilya Ilyich Mechnikov (Elie Metchnikoff) (1845–1916),"
      The Embryo Project Encyclopedia, July 5, 2014.

52   Ibid.

53   *TED*, "Ruairi Robertson: Food for Thought: How Your Belly Controls
      Your Brain," December 7, 2015, video, 14:30.

54   Ibid.

55   Deepak Chopra, "What is the Secret to a Healthy Gut Microbiome?,"
      Chopra, June 7, 2018.

Your microbiome has been helping you since day one. You are protected in your mother's womb, but when you are born, you are exposed to the bacteria around you. With no antibodies and only an innate immune system, what is stopping you from getting sick when first exposed? Through a natural birth, a baby is covered in invisible coats of microorganisms from the mother's birth canal.[56] This initial bacterial colonization helps to promote a stable microbiome for the child.[57] However, a baby delivered by C-section does not get the initial bacteria coatings from the mother's birth canal. It receives its first bacterial coat from a hospital environment, which can contribute to an increased risk of immune deficiencies and bowel diseases later in life.[58] This sparks the controversy over the trend of vaginal seeding, which is when a C-section baby is swabbed with the vaginal fluids of their mother to recreate the natural bacterial transfer.

Your microbiomes have always been on your team, trying to protect you and enhance your overall health. For the gut microbiome to turn on you, you must first go against it. Your diet largely determines the bacterial composition; in order to

56   *TED*, "Ruairi Robertson: Food for Thought: How Your Belly Controls Your Brain," December 7, 2015, video, 14:30.

57   Pearl D. Houghteling and W. Allen Walker, "Why Is Initial Bacterial Colonization of the Intestine Important to Infants' and Children's Health?," *Journal of Pediatric Gastroenterology and Nutrition* 60, no. 3 (March 2015): 294–307; Peter J. Turnbaugh et al., "A Core Gut Microbiome in Obese and Lean Twins," *Nature* 457, no. 7228 (November 30, 2008): 480–84; Jocelyn Spizman, "Allergies, Asthma, and C-sections: The Implications of Birthing Methods," *Exploring Health*, October 20, 2020.

58   Jocelyn Spizman, "Allergies, Asthma, and C-sections: The Implications of Birthing Methods," *Exploring Health*, October 20, 2020.

maintain health, we must preserve the integrity of our gut microbiome. This is important to note for future strategies in treating chronic disease.

I used to watch the cartoon show *Tom and Jerry* when I was a child. Tom is a house cat and Jerry is a mouse, and throughout the show, Tom is constantly chasing Jerry in a comedic way. From this show and common knowledge, I learned at a young age that mice are afraid of cats. Referring back to the show, Jerry was always finding ways to hide and get away from Tom. In a study researching the gut brain relationship, researchers were able to inject the single-celled parasite, Toxoplasma Gondii, which is only capable of reproducing within a cat (the feline family), into mice. [59] Since the parasite can only reproduce inside of a cat, it will die if it were to stay within the mice. Researchers found that when injected into mice, the parasite essentially hijacked the rodent's brain, altering its composition to no longer fear cats (which would increase the parasite's chance of getting inside the cat). [60]

---

59   Global Health, Division of Parasitic Diseases and Malaria, "CDC - Toxoplasmosis - General Information - Frequently Asked Questions (FAQs)," *Centers for Disease Control and Prevention*, last modified September 3, 2020;   Kelly Servick et al., *Brain Parasite May Strip Away Rodents' Fear of Predators-Not Just of Cats*, Science Magazine, January 14, 2020.

60   Ira J. Blader and Jeroen P. Saeij, "Communication between Toxoplasma Gondii and Its Host: Impact on Parasite Growth, Development, Immune Evasion, and Virulence," *Apmis* 117, no. 5–6 (May 2009): 458–76; M. Berdoy et al., "Fatal Attraction in Rats Infected with *Toxoplasma Gondii*," *Royal Society 267*, no. 1452 (August 2000); Justyna Gatkowska et al., "Behavioral Changes in Mice Caused by Toxoplasma Gondii Invasion of Brain." *Parasitology Research 111*, (July 2012): 53–58.

When you have a gut feeling, it is important to be in tune with your body; it may be your gut microbiome trying to communicate with you. Understanding and having a healthy relationship with your gut microbiome could be the key to managing your health.

THREE

INFLAMMATION

———

If you have ever been stung by a bee, you have witnessed the immune system's response to inflammation. Swelling transpires at the site of the bee sting, but the actual work is occurring underneath the skin. In researching why this happens, I stumbled across the work of Dr. Buddy Marterre, a beekeeper and a surgeon in palliative care.[61] What better person to help explain this process?

When a bee first punctures your skin with its stinger, the bee immediately releases melittin, a cytotoxin which affects cells and the immune system.[62] As melittin enters your body, it is on a mission to destroy blood cells, acting as the primary cause of the pain associated with the bee sting.[63]

———

61   Crescendo Interactive Inc, "Dr. William 'Buddy' Marterre Jr. (MDIV'17, P'05) & Ms. Roxanne Marterre (MDIV'17, P'19)," *Wake Forest University: Wake Will Lead*, accessed January 17, 2021.

62   Buddy Marterre, "Bee Stings: Immunology, Allergy, and Treatment," accessed January 17, 2021.

63   Joel Loveridge, "Chemistry of Bees: Bee Stings," *School of Chemistry, University of Bristol*, accessed January 17, 2021.

This is where the immune system, which protects you and keeps you healthy, steps in. As soon as foreign invaders, such as melittin, enter your body, the highly complex immune system works to recognize and, ultimately, destroy it. The first step in providing self-defense is to differentiate proteins that do and do not belong. This is done by your lymphocytes, the white blood cells in the immune system.[64] The energy exerted by our immune system to fight off foreign invaders and produce antibodies for future recognition and destruction may result in swelling, heat, redness, and pain at the site of the sting, in addition to the symptoms from the foreign invader itself.[65] These common symptoms associated with a bee sting are referred to as the "cardinal" signs of inflammation. The original meaning of inflammation is derived from the Latin word "inflammare," which means "to set fire."[66]

All types of cell injury follow a similar sequence of events in order to recover. First, the damaged cells release inflammatory mediators, which results in vasodilation, creating redness and heat. From here, immune cells are recruited to the site of injury, and a leaky endothelium and intracellular fluid shifting lead to edema, swelling caused by trapped fluids. Pain receptors become activated due to swelling and

64 Bruce Alberts et al., *Molecular Biology of the Cell, Fourth Edition* (New York: Garland Science, 2002); Ashley Moor, "Bee Sting: This Is What Happens to Your Body When You Get Stung by a Bee," *BestLife*, May 2, 2019.

65 Buddy Marterre, "Bee Stings: Immunology, Allergy, and Treatment," accessed January 17, 2021.

66 Vocabulary.com, s.v. "inflammation (n.)," accessed January 17, 2021.

inflammatory mediators. The immune cells are able to work, and they restore health in damaged cells.[67]

Inflammation can exist in the short-term, such as a bee sting, and in the long-term, such as chronic illnesses. Acute inflammation is able to resolve itself. Inflammation in the short-term is very beneficial to the body. In order to restore homeostasis in the body, we need inflammatory cascades to react to pathogens and injuries. However, chronic inflammation is very problematic. Notably, acute inflammation responses involve a large physiological scale, while chronic inflammation is typically a low-grade maladaptive response. Occasionally, chronic inflammation goes unnoticed because it progressively takes place over time, so you do not immediately feel or recognize the effects immediately. Harvard Health refers to chronic inflammation as a "fire in your body that you cannot see or feel."[68]

During a short-term inflammatory immune response, like the bee sting example, our bodies are able to fight off this foreign invader and, if you are not allergic, quickly return to a normal state.[69] The removal of foreign invaders is extremely critical for healthy living. Chronic inflammation is the more pressing issue, as the average individual is not aware of the potentially detrimental health effects associated with it. "Your level of chronic inflammation may be very

---

67   Rosário Monteiro and Isabel Azevedo, "Chronic Inflammation in Obesity and the Metabolic Syndrome," *Mediators of Inflammation 2010*, (July 2010): 289645.

68   "Playing with the Fire of Inflammation," *Harvard Health*, October 10, 2019.

69   *Well + Good*, "A Dietitian's Guide to Eating for Inflammation: You Versus Food," November 29, 2019, video, 5:48.

telling of what the future holds for your health," according to Dr. Jane Varner, a family medicine physician at the Palo Alto Medical Foundation.[70]

In chronic inflammation, your immune system is constantly relying upon that army of white blood cells to repair the body.[71] Every time your immune system removes foreign invaders, it also attacks surrounding healthy tissues in your body.[72] With chronic inflammation, the process never stops. You can see the problem here. No wonder chronic inflammation is associated with an increased risk of cardiovascular disease (CVD), diabetes, stroke, neurological disorders (like Alzheimer's), and cancer.[73]

Looking at how our immune system responds to inflammation caused by a bee sting, we can better understand how our bodies react to foods that we eat. We are living in an age where there are new ways to identify, treat, and prevent chronic inflammation. Similar to the venom from a bee sting, some foods (typically processed and refined foods, although there are exceptions, such as red meat, that I will discuss) contain substances that our bodies do not know how to handle, so they will fight against them.[74] When we eat these substances as a normal part of our diet, our immune system responds with a long-term war of chronic inflammation. To prevent this, we need to understand the major contributors

---

70   Ibid.

71   "Playing with the Fire of Inflammation," *Harvard Health*, October 10, 2019.

72   Ibid.

73   *Sutter Health*, "Chronic Inflammation: Impact of Inflammation on Your Body," August 30, 2012, video, 4:02.

74   Ibid.

to this chronic inflammation. We are all in need of a wake-up call. Food may be able to help.

How does our body determine what foods belong or don't belong? There are foods that cause this response, but there also are foods that act against this response. Many foods that cause inflammation are termed "pro-inflammatory," and foods that act against inflammation are termed "anti-inflammatory." In order to explain how pro-inflammatory foods react in the body, we are going to look at two specific pro-inflammatory food triggers: added sugars and red meats.

ADDED SUGARS

Sugar is one of our main energy sources both in the body as glucose and in the diet as carbohydrates. It's important to know the difference between natural and added sugars. They are not synonymous. Certain sugars may present themselves naturally in foods, such as the fructose in fruit and the lactose in milk. A benefit of many natural sugars is that they are often in foods that have fiber and antioxidants.

For the Scientific Reader:

A sugar is a specific type of carbohydrate, a disaccharide, meaning it comprises two monosaccharides. Glucose, fructose, and galactose are the three dietary monosaccharides. The main disaccharides are sucrose (glucose + fructose), lactose (glucose + galactose), and maltose (glucose + glucose). Many people refer to monosaccharides and disaccharides as sugars, but these substances are termed "simple sugars." Dietary sugars are mainly disaccharides. Not all carbohydrates have the same effects as simple sugars.

Added sugars provide little nutritional value, have a high caloric density and are considered to be pro-inflammatory. This means that added sugars provide additional kilocalories without providing additional vitamins and minerals. Our body does not know how to process high levels of sugar at the rate we are eating them in the standard American diet. The average American consumes twenty-two teaspoons of white sugar daily. [75] This is almost three to four times higher than the American Heart Association's (AHA) recommendation of six to nine teaspoons of sugar daily,[76] This recommended sugar intake level is not supposed to be flexible. It is a recommended upper limit, which means that consumption should not exceed this number.

WHY DO WE EAT SO MUCH SUGAR?

Sugar is addicting. When you eat sugar, it activates the sweet taste receptors on your tongue to send a signal to the cerebral cortex in your brain. The cerebral cortex is responsible for processing sensory information from a sweet taste. From here, it activates a rewards system that spans across the entire brain convincing you to eat more sugar, forming your cravings. Dopamine is a neurotransmitter that, when spiked, sends a sense of euphoria to your body, causing cravings. Then, an addiction is born.[77]

The greater your addiction, the less control you have. The food industry is not helping. Almost everything produced

---

75   "Added Sugars on the New Nutrition Facts Label," *FDA*, last modified March 11, 2020.

76   "Added Sugars," American Heart Association, last modified April 17, 2018.

77   *Ted-Ed*, "Nicole Avena: How Sugar Affects the Brain," January 7, 2014, video, 4:53.

today includes sugar. While the sugar content in sweets (like donuts and cookies) is more obvious, sugar can also be found in foods where you might not expect to find it, such as tomato sauce and fruit juices. Why is sugar being added to everything? Manufacturers are adding sugar to give foods a sweeter flavor, a better texture, a more appealing color, and more preservatives to last longer. It's no wonder that sugary products sell so well.[78] The more sugar that is available, the more you consume, the more you crave, and the more that is produced. It is a vicious cycle.

DIABETES

Diabetes mellitus, or just diabetes, is a metabolic disease that causes high blood sugar. Type I diabetes is an autoimmune disorder where the body attacks and ultimately halts the production of insulin. Most people who have type I were diagnosed earlier in life. On the other hand, type II diabetes occurs when the body cannot produce enough insulin and/ or the body does not respond appropriately to insulin due to poor diet choices. The rates of type II diabetes have continued to grow throughout the years.[79] We are overworking our beta cells, which are found in the pancreas and are responsible for producing insulin. Anytime you eat sugar, the beta cells recruit insulin to manage the sugar. Insulin converts the sugar into usable energy and feeds it to the muscles and liver.

---

78   Kara R. Goldfein et al., "Why Sugar Is Added to Food: Food Science 101," *Comprehensive Reviews in Food Science and Food Safety* 14, no. 5 (August 3, 2015): 644–56.

79   "Diabetes: Rates of New Diagnosed Cases of Type 1 and Types 2 Diabetes Continue to Rise Among Children, Teens," *Centers for Disease Control and Prevention*, last modified February 11, 2020.

For the Scientific Reader:

All sugars are carbohydrates. When you eat carbohydrates, the body is constantly trying to break larger sugars down into the simplest form of sugar, glucose, to provide energy for your body and brain. The brain is primarily dependent on glucose as an energy source.[80]

At the rate we are eating sugar, there are not enough places for it to go, forcing insulin to store sugar as fat.[81] The more energy the beta cells exert, the more tired they get. Our beta cells are overworked, which can cause them to wear down. If we continue on this path, beta cells might not be able to work at all eventually, thus no insulin will be able to be made. This results in type II diabetes.[82] According to the Centers for Disease Control and Prevention (CDC), "more than thirty-four million Americans have diabetes, about one in ten, and approximately 90–95 percent of them have type 2 diabetes."[83]

INFLAMMATORY

Added sugars are pro-inflammatory. We need inflammation in order to heal; when we get stung by a bee, we rely on our

80   Jacqueline Fung, "Nutrient and Health - Carbohydrates: Sugars," *Food Safety Focus*, last modified November 16, 2018.

81   Kamal Patel, "How Are Carbohydrates Converted into Fat Deposits?," *Examine*, last modified February 1, 2013.

82   *TEDx Talks*, "Jody Stanislaw: Sugar is Not a Treat," December 12, 2017, video, 15:31.

83   U.S. Department of Health & Human Services, "Diabetes: Type 2 Diabetes," *Centers for Disease Control and Prevention (CDC)*, last modified May 30, 2019.

immune system and inflammatory cascades to return us to health. However, being in a constant state of inflammation is detrimental to our health. When sugar combines with fats and proteins in your bloodstream, Advanced Glycation End products (AGEs) are created endogenously. AGEs can also be found in the blood due to exogenous sources, such as consuming foods that are high in AGEs. AGEs are an inflammatory biomarker, meaning that the level of AGEs found in your body can be a good estimate for measuring inflammation.[84]

If you have ever noticed a worsened complexion in a high sugar diet, it is because AGEs break down collagen.[85] Collagen is the most abundant protein in your body and a major component of healthy skin.[86] A reason why you get wrinkles as you age is because your body produces less collagen throughout time.[87] Collagen is not just a key component in skin, but in your joints, as well. The more sugar you eat, the more collagen is destroyed, and therefore the harder it is for your joints to recover. Cutaneous abnormalities, medical conditions that affect the integumentary system (which encompasses the skin, hair, nails, and linked muscles), are

84   RS Pinto et al., "Advanced Glycation End Products as Biomarkers for Cardiovascular Disease: Browning Clarifying Atherogenesis," *Biomarkers in Medicine 14*, no. 8 (June 2020).

85   Gion Fessel et al., "Advanced Glycation End-Products Reduce Collagen Molecular Sliding to Affect Collagen Fibril Damage Mechanisms but Not Stiffness," *Plos One*, November 3, 2014.

86   "Abundant Protein," *International Journal of Applied Biology and Pharmaceutical Technology*, accessed February 15, 2021.

87   Ruta Ganceviciene et al., "Skin Anti-Aging Strategies," *Dermato-Endocrinology 4*, no. 3 (July 2012): 308–19.

rooted in that low-grade chronic inflammation. Diets low in dietary AGEs may be beneficial.[88] In fact, spices like cinnamon and oregano have shown inhibition properties toward fructose-induced AGE formation.[89] Increased levels of AGEs have also been associated with worsened progression of degenerative diseases, such as Alzheimer's, diabetes, and atherosclerosis.[90] Certain types of fats, like saturated and trans fats, are typically known to be the enemy of atherosclerosis due to its effects on cholesterol. I will discuss this more in-depth in the fats chapter. Unfortunately, many people are misinformed that sugar is to blame just as much as saturated and trans fats. Atherosclerosis is a disease where the arterial walls are narrowed and/or blocked, which can result in high blood pressure, blood clots, and eventually cardiovascular disease (CVD). While fat causes an excess build-up of bad cholesterol (which gets lodged in the arterial walls), sugar causes the arterial wall itself to become stiff, which builds resistance against blood flow.[91]

---

88   F. William Danby, "Nutrition and Aging Skin: Sugar and Glycation," *Clinics in Dermatology 28*, no. 4 (July-August 2010): 409–411.

89   Ibid.

90   Sheldon Rowan et al., "Mechanistic Targeting of Advanced Glycation End-Products in Age-Related Diseases," *Bichimica et Biophysica Act (BBA) – Molecular Basis of Disease 1864*, no. 12 (December 2018): 3631–3643; Serena Del Turco and Giuseppina Basta, "An Update on Advanced Glycation Endproducts and Athersclerosis," *BioFactors 38*, no. 4 (2012): 266–274.

91   *Thomas* DeLaur "What Sugar Does to Your Brain & Body: The Truth About Sugar," January 22, 2018, video, 7:10.

For the Scientific Reader:

The presence of many compounds similar in nature to AGEs increases in the body as a result of consuming excess added sugar. Pro-inflammatory cytokines, which are signaling molecules that promote inflammation, are a potential problem as you exceed the upper limit on sugars recommended by the AHA. Cytokines have an inconsistent nomenclature, often being referred to as interleukins.[92] The three main pro-inflammatory cytokines are tumor necrosis factor (TNF), interleukin six (IL-6), and interleukin eight (IL-8).[93]

TNF helps the body attack foreign invaders and heal damaged tissues, making it an essential part of the immune system in healthy individuals. However, excess levels of TNF, a consequence of added sugars, can lead to inflammation. IL-6 plays an important role in the transition between acute and chronic inflammation. IL-6 actually has a dual effect. It can provide defense responses in short-term inflammation and pro-inflammatory consequences in long-term, chronic inflammation.[94] IL-6 has been recognized

---

92   José Noel Ibrahim et al., "Cytokine Signatures in Hereditary Fever Syndromes (HFS)," *Cytokine & Growth Factor Reviews* 33 (February 2017): 19–34.

93   Shinwan Kany et al., "Cytokines in Inflammatory Disease," *International Journal of Molecular Sciences* 20, no. 23 (November 28, 2019): 6008; *Thomas DeLauer*, "Carbs and Inflammation: How Sugar Causes Inflammation," August 1, 2017, video, 5:29.

94   *Thomas DeLauer*, "Carbs and Inflammation: How Sugar Causes Inflammation," August 1, 2017, video, 5:29.

for its pro-inflammatory associations and links to cardiovascular disease and cancer since 1990.[95] IL-6 is similar to IL-8 since both are major mediators of inflammatory responses.[96] IL-8 attracts neutrophils (the most abundant white blood cells found in the circulatory system) in inflammatory regions. Neutrophils are only beneficial to a certain extent; then, they are linked to the progression of inflammation, with evidence linked to cancer.[97]

TNF proteins circulate in the blood and trigger inflammatory processes at target areas by prompting the production of IL-6 immune system molecules involved in driving inflammation by destroying cartilage and bone.[98] IL-6 and IL-8 are cytokines produced during the inflammatory response: "In autoimmune diseases, IL-6 not only maintains inflammation, but also modifies the immune responses."[99] IL-6 adopts a dangerous role in leukocyte recruitment and cell accumulation at the site of injury in chronic inflammation, which may provide the basis of amplification

95   Michel Jourdan et al., "Constitutive Production of Interleukin-6 and Immunologic Features in Cardiac Myxomas," *Arthritis & Rheumatism* 33, no. 3 (March 1990): 398–402; Shinwan Kany et al., "Cytokines in Inflammatory Disease," *International Journal of Molecular Sciences* 20, no. 23 (November 28, 2019): 6008.

96   Ibid.

97   Lingyun Wu et al., "Tumor-Associated Neutrophils in Cancer: Going Pro," *Cancers* 11, no. 4 (2019): 564.

98   Ibid,

99   Cem Gabay, "Interleukin-6 and Chronic Inflammation," *Arthritis Research & Therapy* 8, no. 2 (July 28, 2006).

in chronic inflammatory proliferation. One of the main differences between IL-6 and IL-8 is that IL-8 has a longer half-life.[100] Unlike other cytokines, IL-8 attracts neutrophils, a major population of immigrant cells in periodontal (gum) disease.[101]

TABLE SUGAR AND HFCS

The two most common added sugars are table sugar, also known as sucrose, and high-fructose corn syrup (HFCS). Both table sugar and HFCS consist of glucose and fructose sugar molecules; however, their ratios differ. The composition within table sugar is exactly 50:50 glucose:fructose, while HFCS is typically 42:55, containing more fructose than glucose.[102]

Table sugar and HFCS can easily be broken down into glucose and fructose to be distributed throughout the body. The body is more capable of handling complex carbohydrates because it has time to release insulin and other blood glucose regulatory hormones, like glucagon, which can add or remove glucose to the bloodstream when necessary. [103] Not giving the body adequate time to release insulin at the

---

100 Ibid.

101 M. Bickel, "The role of interleukin-8 in inflammation and mechanisms of regulation," *Journal of Periodontology* vol. 64, no. 5 (May 1993): 456–60.

102 Kamal Patel, "What is the Difference Between High Fructose Corn Syrup (HFCS) and Sugar?," *Examine*, last modified January 13, 2020.

103 *The Source Chiropractor*, "How Sugar Leads to Pain and Inflammation," October 7, 2016, video: 3:50; "The Functions of Carbohydrates in the Body," *The European Food Information Council (EUFIC)*, last modified January 14, 2020.

appropriate rates results in a backup in your beta cells, which, if prolonged, will lead to type II diabetes.

Both table sugar and HFCS contain fructose. Most people are confused by this concept. Table sugar and HFCS are bad for you, but fruits are good for you. Yet, both contain fructose. How is this possible? Fructose is considered to be the sweetest of all the sugars. Even though it has the same chemical formula as glucose, it has a different chemical structure.[104] Interestingly, the body responds to fructose differently when processed in forms other than fruits, such as a high concentration in HFCS. It is extremely challenging to consume a surplus of fructose from whole fruits, whereas added sugars, such as table sugar and HFCS, are more highly concentrated in fructose.

For the Scientific Reader:

Glucose may be stored as glycogen, which limits the amount in the bloodstream that eventually turns into fat. On the other hand, fructose is almost exclusively metabolized in the liver. A larger proportion of "diet-derived fructose than glucose metabolites are available for conversion to fat."[105]

When you consume table sugar and HFCS, you are not just consuming fructose, but glucose, too. When we think about added sugars, we must think about glucose and fructose acting together.

---

104 Jacqueline Fung, "Nutrient and Health - Carbohydrates: Sugars," *Food Safety Focus*, last modified November 16, 2018.

105 Sarah A. Hannou et al., "Fructose Metabolism and Metabolic Disease," *The Journal of Clinical Investigation 128*, no. 2 (February 2018): 545–555.

The rise in added sugar consumption over the past decades has been a major contributor to disease. Table sugar, HFCS, and other added sugars are high in calories, per gram, compared to other food components, but adding them to foods provides only energy and little to no nutrients; this is referred to as "empty" calories.[106] Consuming added sugars increases not only your risk of obesity, but other serious illnesses, as well. Since 2016, cancer research has been able to link tumor growth in breast cancer with fructose from added sugars, such as table sugar and HFCS.[107] Fructose in HFCS has also been associated with lung metastasis, the spread of breast cancer to the lungs.

Studies have shown a diminished production of nitric oxide due to increased fructose consumption.[108] Nitric oxide is an essential vasodilator, relaxing the muscles of your blood

---

106   Rudy Mawer, "6 Reasons Why High-Fructose Corn Syrup Is Bad for You," *Healthline*, September 27, 2019.

107   Samir Faruque et al., "The Dose Makes the Poison: Sugar and Obesity in the United States – A Review," *Polish Journal of Food and Nutrition Sciences 69*, no. 3 (2019): 219–233; Jordan W. Strober and Matthew J. Brady, "Dietary Fructose Consumption and Triple-Negative Breast Cancer Incidence," *Frontiers in Endocrinology* 10 (June 12, 2019); Honor Whiteman, "Study Links High Sugar Intake to Increased Risk of Breast Cancer," *MedicalNewsToday*, January 4, 2016; Rolaynne Kimmons, "Sugar in Western Diets Increases Risk for Breast Cancer Tumor and Metastasis," *The University of Texas MD Anderson Cancer Center*, December 31, 2015.

108   Alice Victoria Klein and Hosen Kiat, "The Mechanisms Underlying Fructose-Induced Hypertension: A Review," *Journal of Hypertension 33*, no. 5 (February 2015): 912–920.

vessels, and it is produced by almost every cell in the body.[109] To ensure good blood vessel health, you must have adequate levels of nitric oxide to increase blood flow and lower blood pressure, which is critical to your heart and cardiovascular health. By consuming too much fructose, we are putting our cardiovascular health at risk.

Dr. Willian Davis, a cardiologist and the author of *Wheat Belly,* describes people as "boiling pots of inflammation: hot, steaming, churning cauldrons of disordered, chaotic inflammatory responses." This vivid description stems from the excessive amounts of sugar in our diets. The worst part is that we do not even realize it.[110]

Many experts believe that added sugars, such as table sugar and HFCS, are key factors in today's obesity epidemic and chronic inflammation.[111] The average American is eating way too many added sugars. These high consumption rates of added sugars can help explain our country's extensive health problems and dependence on medicine. While sugar can be beneficial to your body in moderation, as a primary energy source, excess sugar can pose detrimental health effects stemming from inflammation. Today, added sugars can be found in almost any food item. Keep an eye out for the amounts of

---

109   Vikas Kapil et al., "Dietary Nitrate Provides Sustained Blood Pressure Lowering in Hypertensive Patients," *American Heart Association: Hypertension 65*, no. 2 (February 2015): 320–7.

110   "The Silent Killer," *Trivita*, accessed January 18, 2021.

111   Robert H Lustig et al., "Public Health: The Toxic Truth About Sugar," *Nature 482*, no. 7383 (2012): 27–29; George A Bray et al., "Consumption of High-Fructose Corn Syrup in Beverages May Play A Role in the Epidemic of Obesity," *The American Journal of Clinical Nutrition 79*, no. 4 (2004): 537–543.

added sugars on nutrition labels. The American Heart Association recommends no more than twenty-four and thirty-six grams of added sugar for women and men, respectively.[112] To put this in perspective, Oreos contain fourteen grams of added sugars, and a serving size is only three cookies. If you are a woman and eat six Oreo cookies, you are already over the recommended added sugar consumption for the day. To give another example of a food where added sugars may be hidden, Ocean Spray Cran-Grape juice contains twenty-two grams of added sugars per cup. One cup is considered to be eight fluid ounces; if you use glasses that hold ten fluid ounces, you are already over the daily recommended added sugar consumption. It is that easy; no wonder it is such a problem.

We have all heard the common saying from Mary Poppins, "A spoonful of sugar helps the medicine go down." Dr. Lance von Stade proves truthfulness in this saying by explaining that increased sugar consumption will cause harm to your overall health, which will force you to depend on more medicine.[113]

RED MEATS

It is quite simple—red meat is more harmful for us than we think. As evidenced by a multitude of clinical studies, consuming red meat can have negative health ramifications, primarily due to its pro-inflammatory properties.[114]

---

112   "Added Sugar in the Diet," *Harvard Health*, accessed February 15, 2021.

113   Ibid.

114   Jukka Montonen et al., "Consumption of Red Meat and Whole-Grain Bread in Relation to Biomarkers of Obesity, Inflammation, Glucose Metabolism and Oxidative Stress," *European Journal of Nutrition* 52, no. 1 (February 2013): 337–45.

While avoiding meat is advised if you are struggling with an existing health concern, it's not easy to eliminate since animal proteins undoubtedly remain a central aspect of food traditions in many cultures. Therefore, this chapter aims to provide tips and tricks on how to prepare red meat in "healthier" ways that can mitigate some of its harmful components.

INFLAMMATORY BIOMARKERS

Animal products naturally contain specific pro-inflammatory compounds that can be detrimental to our health. Associations between red meat consumption and increased inflammatory biomarkers have been noted.[115] These biomarkers included C reactive proteins (CRP).[116]

For the Scientific Reader:

CRP is synthesized by the liver cells (hepatocytes), and they are sent to the bloodstream under conditions of inflammation.[117] Adequate amounts of CRP exhibit beneficial anti-inflammatory characteristics by activating phagocytic cells to help recognize and remove foreign pathogens, which are considered

---

115   Ibid.

116   Ying-yi Luan and Yong-ming Yao, "The Clinical Significance and Potential Role of C-Reactive Protein in Chronic Inflammatory and Neurodegenerative Disease," *Frontiers in Immunology*, no. 9 (June 2018): 1302.

117   Ibid.

to be anti-inflammatory characteristics.[118] Unfortunately, this process may become indicative of a disease when it is activated by autoantibodies such as in immune thrombocytopenic purpura (ITP), an autoimmune disease where blood doesn't clot normally.[119]

High levels of CRP can worsen tissue damage by increasing pro-inflammatory cytokines, a signaling molecule that precipitates an inflammatory cascade.[120] According to the Mayo Clinic, standard levels of CRP are less than 10 mg/L, whereas elevated CRP levels are indicative of underlying medical conditions.[121] Consistently high levels of CRP may

---

118   Maarten Jungen et al., "Inflammatory Biomarkers in Patieents with Sciatica: A Systematic Review," *BMS Musculoskeletal Disorders 20*, no. 1 (April 9, 2019):156; Ying-yi Luan and Yong-ming Yao, "The Clinical Significance and Potential Role of C-Reactive Protein in Chronic Inflammatory and Neurodegenerative Disease," *Frontiers in Immunology*, no. 9 (June 2018): 1302.

119   Sara M. Nehring et al., "C Reactive Protein," StatPearls, *U.S. National Library of Medicine*, June 5, 2020.

120   Nicole E Kramer et al., "A Clinical Model for Identifying an Inflammatory Phenotype in Mood Disorders," *J Psychiatr Res 113*, (February 2019):148–158; Sara M. Nehring et al., "C Reactive Protein," StatPearls, *U.S. National Library of Medicine*, June 5, 2020.

121   Mayo Clinic Staff, "C-Reactive Protein Test," *Mayo Clinic*, November 21, 2017; Alexander Landry et al., "Causes and Outcomes of Markedly Elevated C-Reactive Protein Levels," *Official Publication of The College of Family Physicians of Canada 63*, 3 (June 2017): e316–e323.

result in cardiovascular diseases.[122] What does this mean? How much red meat consumption is acceptable? The World Cancer Research Fund explains the importance of finding a happy medium for meat eaters. Meat can be a valuable nutrient source, but you must keep in mind that overabundant consumption is associated with inflammation and increased disease risk. While it is hard to give exact recommended levels of how much meat you should or should not be eating since many factors may alter this amount, the World Cancer Research Fund determined that if you eat red meat, you should limit consumption to just three portions each week; one portion is considered to be about 350–500 grams.[123] Processed meat is correlated with elevated CRP levels compared to lean red meat. The World Cancer Research fund recommends individuals completely cut out their consumption of processed meats. While lean and unprocessed red meats may be considered "better" for you than processed meats, they are still associated with increased health risks and a negative relationship with inflammation.[124]

---

122 Carl Nathan and Aihao Ding, "Nonresolving Inflammation," *Cell Press 140*, no. 6 (March 2010): 871–882.

123 "Limit Red and Processed Meat," *World Cancer Research Fund International*, accessed February 23, 2021.

124 Tianying Wu et al., "Unprocessed Red Meat Intakes are Associated with increased Inflammation, Triglycerides and HDL Cholesterol in Past Smokers." *Nutrition & Dietetics 77*, no. 2 (June 2019): 182–188; Sylvia H. Ley et al., "Associations Between Red Meat and Biomarkers of Inflammation and Glucose Metabolism in Women." *The American Journal of Clinical Nutrition 99*, no. 2 (February 2014): 352–360.

Fortunately, there is sufficient evidence that a healthful diet can reduce the negative consequences from inflammatory molecules. Epidemiological studies have estimated that whole grains reduce CRP levels by 7 percent![125] In a specific study looking at young, healthy women, consuming over one serving of whole grains daily was associated with a lower risk of elevated CRP levels.[126] The specific amount of whole grains required for optimum CRP reduction is not yet defined. Whole grains are thought to be anti-inflammatory in nature because of their synergistic activity with some health-promoting compounds, e.g., dietary fiber and antioxidants. We will explore other human health benefits of whole grains in the succeeding chapter.

TMAO

In addition to the association with pro-inflammatory bio-markers, clinicians also discourage the consumption of red meat because of its carnitine and choline content.[127]

While carnitine and choline contribute positively to overall health, both dietary nutrients have been linked to elevated trimethylamine oxide (TMAO), a

---

125 Michael Lefevre and Satya Jonnalagadda, "Effect of Whole Grains on Markers of Subclinical Inflammation," *Nutrition Reviews 70*, no. 7 (May 22, 2012): 387–96.

126 Audrey J. Gaskins et al., "Whole Grains are Associated with Serum Concentrations of High Sensitivity C-Reactive Protein among Premenopausal Women," *The Journal of Nutrition 140*, no. 9 (September 2010): 1669–1676.

127 Zeneg Wang et al., "Gut Flora Metabolism of Phosphatidylcholine Promotes Cardiovascular Disease," *Nature 472*, no. 7341 (April 2011): 57–63.

pro-inflammatory metabolite associated with cardiovascular diseases.[128] Choline, specifically, produces trimethylamine (TMA), which converts to TMAO in the liver. Your diet can change the composition of the microorganisms within your gut microbiome. When you consistently eat red meat, your body will produce more microbes that are able to metabolize the meat. These microbes will produce more and more TMA and, therefore, TMAO, as you continue to eat red meat, elevating your TMAO levels.[129] Dr. Robert Lustig, an endocrinologist describes TMAO to be the stickiest, most inflammatory substance that we have in our bodies."[130] Although the kidney filters TMAO out of the blood, it can accumulate in the body and increase the risk of cardiovascular diseases (CVD). If you consume a lot of red meat, cardiologists highly recommend their patients get their blood tested to look at their TMAO levels and predict their CVD risk.[131] If you find out your levels of TMAO are high, take a deep breath. You can reverse elevated TMAO levels by stopping or significantly decreasing your red meat consumption.

AGES

Diets that include red meats contain high levels of AGEs. Reports of inflammatory biomarkers, such as CRP

---

128 Xiao-Hua Yu et al., "Foam Cells in Atherosclerosis," *Clinica Chimica Acta 424*, (September 2013): 245–252.

129 "Red Meat, TMAO, and Your Heart," *Harvard Health*, September 2019.

130 *University of California Television*, "Red Meat, Disease, and Inflammation," August 7, 2020, video, 4:31.

131 Joel Kahn, "TMAO: What We Eat and What's Eating Us," Dr. Joel Kahn, *Huffington Post*, July 11, 2016.

correlate with AGEs in the blood (refer to the added sugars section to review more on AGEs).[132] Yet, most people are unaware of AGEs, how they work, and why they are harmful. Chances are if you regularly eat foods that have been exposed to high temperatures through grilling, charring, and baking, you are likely exposed to many AGEs. Many foods naturally contain AGEs; however, specific food items, such as animal-derived products, are especially high in AGEs.

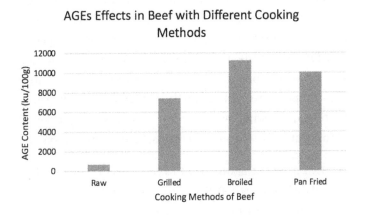

Figure 1: AGEs Effect in Beef with Different Cooking Methods.[133]

132 *Whitney E. RD.* "The Truth About Meat + Inflammation," May 14, 2019, video, 6:20.

133 Seppo Pussa, "Dietary Advanced Glycation End Products," *Acne Einstein*, accessed on February 15, 2021; IOS Press BV, "New Study Postulates the Role of Dietary Advanced Glycation End Products in the Risk of Alzheimer's Disease," *ScienceDaily*, February 3, 2015; Heejung An, "Comparison of AGEs Produced by Different Cooking Methods," *Nongshim R&D*, November 8, 2013.

You can see this reaction when your meats turn brown![134] When you increase dietary AGEs and they accumulate in the body, they can disrupt normal cell function.[135] These compounds accumulate significantly in the body causing oxidative stress, chronic inflammation, and increasing the overall risk of chronic disease.[136] While our bodies exhibit antioxidant and enzymatic activity to eliminate AGEs, consistently consuming red meat strains our bodily functions such that we cannot keep up with the level of AGEs coming in.[137]

While the most effective solution to reduce AGE levels in your body is to eliminate or limit consumption of foods known to elevate AGE levels, promising evidence suggests alternative options may allow you to continue enjoying your favorite foods in moderation. As mentioned before, high-temperature cooking methods such as grilling, frying, toasting, or roasting causes the level of AGEs to skyrocket. If you are going to consume red meats, then try high-moisture

134 Heejung An, "Comparison of AGEs Produced by Different Cooking Methods," *Nongshim R&D*, November 8, 2013; "Health Warning for High-Heat Meat," *Hospital and Healthcare*, September 8, 2020.

135 "Health Warning for High-Heat Meat," *Hospital and Healthcare*, September 8, 2020.

136 Jaime Uribarri et al., "Circulating Glycotoxins and Dietary Advanced Glycation Endproducts: Two Links to Inflammatory Response, Oxidative Stress, and Aging," *J Gerontol A Biol Sci Med Sci 62*, 4 (April 2007): 427–33.

137 Xinle Wu and Vincent M. Monnier, "Enzymatic Deglycation of Proteins," *Arch Biochem Biophys 419*, no. 1 (November 2003): 16–24; James R. Connor et al., "Some Clues as to the Regulation, Expression, Function, and Distribution of Fructosamine-3-Kinase and Fructosamine-3-Kinase-Related Protein," *Ann N Y Acad Sci 1043*, (June 2005): 824–36.

cooking techniques with lower heat. For example, marinating your meat in acidic marinades not only adds more flavor, but can actually inhibit the formation of AGEs. New research reported that less than half the amounts of AGEs were produced when beef was marinated with a mixture of lemon juice and vinegar compared to meat that was not marinated.[138]

MARINADES

Many people report feeling sick after consuming red meat. Why? Is it the saturated fat or the AGEs intake? Another likely culprit is that we do not have enough hydrochloric acid in our stomachs to digest the high levels of protein from red meat. This often causes digestive discomfort because our bodies are not equipped to regularly digest such complex proteins. [139]

One effective remedy is to marinade your meat before consuming it. Acidic ingredients in marinades, such as lemon juice, vinegar, and wine can help to denature those long proteins. The marinades help do the dirty work by aiding in the catabolism (breakdown) of proteins to amino acids so that your stomach enzymes are not overworked. Apple cider vinegar (ACV) works as a great marinade as it introduces more acid into the digestive track, and certain types of ACV contain yeast and bacteria from fermentation; this

---

138 Jamie Uribarri et al., "Advanced Glycation End Products in Foods and a Practical Guide to Their Reduction in the Diet," *Journal of the American Dietetic Association 110*, no. 6 (June 2010): 911–16.e1.

139 Julie Bender-Sibbio, "Could Hypochlorydria Be at the Root of Your Digestive Problems?," *JBS Nutrition and Wellness* (blog), November 28, 2017.

murky solution is referred to as the "mother," which contains minerals and probiotics that promote gut health.[140] Interestingly, certain fruits may also act as great marinades. Pineapple, kiwi, fig, and mango contain an enzyme called protease that plays an important role in tenderizing meat, breaking down meat fibers and softening it to make it more palatable.[141] Next time you pick-up a steak from the butcher, try adding acidic marinade for a flavorful dish—without the stomach cramps!

SATURATED FAT

Modern diets worldwide contain large quantities of red meats, such as steak and hamburger. The leading countries for meat consumption are the US, Australia, and Argentina.[142] If you compare cattle in the US to Argentina, you will immediately notice a difference. Argentinian cattle are predominately grass-fed, while US cattle are fed a corn-based diet. This results in US beef having higher saturated fat levels than beef in Argentina. Corn consists of highly branched amino acids, like Leucine, Isoleucine, and Valine. An amino acid group must be removed in order to convert corn into usable energy, thereby resulting in a fatty accumulation in the liver. Grain-fed cattle, such as from a corn-based diet, contains higher levels of saturated fats

---

140 Kiara Anthony, "How to Increase Stomach Acid at Home," *Healthline*, March 7, 2019.

141 "Fruit Enzymes Tenderise Meat," *Science Learning Hub*, accessed February 24, 2021.

142 Hannah Ritchie and Max Roser, "Meat and Dairy Production," *Our World in Data*, last modified November 2019.

than grass-fed cattle.[143] This byproduct is why American beef looks visibly fattier than grass-fed beef and contains higher levels of saturated fat.[144]

Even if all the cattle in the world were grass-fed, the level of saturated fats found in red meat would still pose an issue. Naturally, red meats contain high levels of saturated fat. Different cuts of beef contain different levels of saturated fat. A ribeye steak has ten grams of saturated fat per one hundred grams. This is almost at the upper limit of daily saturated fat intake! The AHA recommends a consumption of saturated fat to make up no more than 5 to 6 percent of your daily calories. For a person who follows a two-thousand-calorie diet, this would be about 120 calories (thirteen grams).[145] The USDA defines lean red meat as having less than 4.5 grams of saturated fat.[146] Try to substitute a ribeye steak for a sirloin tip steak, the leanest cut with around 1.6 grams of saturated fat per one hundred grams.

For the Scientific Reader:

Diets high in saturated fats are known to cause endotoxemia, an accumulation of endotoxins/ lipo-polysaccharides found on the outer membrane of gram-negative bacteria, and result in the gut

---

143   Cynthia A Daley et al., "A Review of Fatty Acid Profiles and Antioxidant Content in Grass-Fed and Grain-Fed Beef," *Nutrition Journal* 9, no. 10 (March 2010).

144   *University of California Television*, "Red Meat, Disease, and Inflammation," August 7, 2020, video, 4:31.

145   "Saturated Fat," *American Heart Association*, accessed February 23, 2021.

146   Mayo Clinic Staff, "Cuts of Beef: A Guide to the Leanest Selections," *Mayo Clinic*, October 29, 2019.

microbiome absorbing toxins found in food that is typically able to be blocked, failing to protect the body.[147]

Saturated fats are also associated with increasing levels of your bad cholesterol, low-density lipoprotein, which may result in atherosclerosis and cardiovascular disease. Interestingly, a reason as to why a diet high in saturated fats may increase your risk of obesity is because saturated fats cause inflammation within adipose tissues which is an early sign of obesity. In obesity, macrophages, a type of white blood cell, are accumulated in adipose tissues.[148]

All of these factors contribute to the inflammatory characteristics of saturated fats. Short-term, inflammatory cascades will occur to repair damaged cells, but long-term, this inflammation may be the main culprit of metabolic syndromes, conditions to increase the risk of diabetes, heart diseases, and strokes. [149]

Side note:

Saturated fats are also found naturally in dairy products. However, because the chemical composition is distinct to that of animal proteins, the body processes

---

147 Begoña Ruiz-Núññz et al., "The Relation of Saturated Fatty Acids with Low-Grade Inflammation and Cardiovascular Disease," *The Journal of Nutritional Biochemistry 36*, (October 2016): 1–20.

148 Ibid.

149 Chumjit Bui et al., "Acute Effect of a Single High-fat Meal on Forearm Blood Flow, Blood Pressure and Heart Rate in Healthy Male Asians and Causasians: A Pilot Study," *Southeast Asian Journal of Tropical Medicine and Public Health 41*, no. 2 (March 2010): 490–500.

it differently, resulting in a unique physiological response. I will discuss saturated fats in greater detail in the Fats chapter.

Like the bee sting, many foods can trigger inflammatory responses in the body. While chronic inflammation caused by nutrient deficiencies may be harder to spot compared to the acute bee sting example, understanding low-grade chronic inflammation and identifying universal and personal pro-inflammatory food triggers may be the key to restoring your relationship with your gut microbiome and living a healthy life.

TWO

PRINCIPLES OF THE FOOD-CAN-HEAL MINDSET

FOUR

GLUTEN AND GRAINS

Everywhere you look, people are going gluten-free. People often think, "A gluten-free diet is healthier." "It makes me feel better." "I will lose weight." The science behind these claims is scant at best. For example, people associate a gluten-free diet with weight loss; no scientifically proven studies have revealed that a gluten-free diet is associated with weight loss. Gluten can make foods palatable, and without it, sugars and fats are needed to cover them up. If you are curious, compare the nutrition label of a gluten-free snack with its gluten-containing counterpart. You may notice an increased percentage differences in saturated fats and added sugars in some of the gluten-free versions.

HERE IS WHAT YOU NEED TO KNOW ABOUT BOING GLUTEN-FREE

According to Joseph Murray, a gastroenterologist at the Mayo Clinic, approximately one percent of Americans have celiac disease, an autoimmune condition in which the presence of gluten causes damage to the small intestine.[150] For people who suffer from celiac disease, gluten is toxic; however, this does not indicate that gluten is toxic or even unhealthy to others. Eliminating gluten from your diet can be dangerous. Foods that contain gluten also contain essential nutrients.

This hasn't stopped the growing popularity of going gluten-free. Between the years of 2009 to 2014, the reported gluten-free diet population tripled (0.5 to 1.7 percent), while the prevalence of those who suffered from celiac disease remained the same.[151] In 2019, the global gluten-free market was estimated at around $21.61 billion, and once again the percentage of people suffering from celiac disease remained relatively the same.[152] The global gluten-free market is expected to reach $36 billion by 2026.[153] The director of the Celiac Disease Center at Columbia University, Peter H. R.

---

150 *Mayo Clinic*, "Mayo Clinic Minute: The Truth About Gluten," December 14, 2015, video, 1:07.

151 Rok Seon Choung et al., "Less Hidden Celiac Disease but Increased Gluten Avoidance Without A Diagnosis in the USA: Findings from the National Health and Nutrition Examination Surveys from 2009 to 2014," *Mayo Clinic Proceedings*, (December 2016): 30634-6.

152 "Gluten-Free Products Market Size, Share & Trends Analyst Report By Product (Bakery Products, Dairy/Dairy Alternatives), By Distribution Channel (Grocery Stores, Mass Merchandiser), By Region, And Segment Forecasts, 2020-2027," *Grand View Research*, February 2020.

153 "Global Gluten Free Products (Food) Market Size Will Reach USD 36 Billion by 2026: Facts & Factors," *GlobeNewswire*, accessed February 15, 2021.

Green, MD, stated that going gluten-free is a "trendy diet."[154] Dr. Green wrote a book on gluten called *Gluten Exposed* that I encourage you to check out if you want to learn more about his research and the risks of following a gluten-free diet by those without an intolerance.[155]

It is common for people who experience chronic indigestion to accuse gluten as the culprit for their discomfort. Yet, this is much more unlikely than one might think. It is never in your best interest to self-diagnose a gluten sensitivity. Misdiagnosing yourself with gluten intolerance can lead to vitamin deficiencies, a shortage of fiber, and even weight gain due to the added sugars and fats for taste in gluten-free foods.

It is highly recommended to consult your doctor if you believe you have a gluten sensitivity. Even if your indigestion issues start to resolve on a gluten-free diet, it does not mean that you have a gluten sensitivity. The odds of being more sensitive to specific carbohydrates in wheat are greater than your odds of being sensitive to gluten itself. Thus, gluten is more of a scapegoat than a culprit of digestive discomfort. If this applies to you, have you ever considered that it was not the gluten protein itself that is making you sick? Ask your doctor about fermentable oligosaccharides, disaccharides, monosaccharides, and polyols, or the easier version to say, FODMAPs.

---

154   Kathleen Doheny, "What's Behind the Gluten-Free Trend?," *WebMD Health News*, September 16, 2016.

155   Peter H. R. Green and Rory Jones, *Gluten Exposed: The Science Behind the Hype and How to Navigate to a Healthy, Symptom-Free Life* (New York: William Morrow and Company, 2016).

For the Scientific Reader:
Carbohydrates are generally absorbed as they pass through the small intestines. FODMAPs are a group of short-chain carbohydrates that may be inadequately absorbed (this is similar to fiber, which we will be discussing shortly).[156] When FODMAPs reach the colon (which contains billions of bacteria), excess hydrogen (and other gases) is produced as the bacteria ferments FODMAPs as a source of energy.[157] This will typically lead to symptoms such as bloating, gas, cramps, constipation, and/or diarrhea.[158]

Jessica Biesiekierski, a registered nutritionist and researcher of dietetics and human nutrition, believes FODMAPs, and not gluten, more likely explain the food intolerance many people experience. She studied gluten sensitivities within non-celiac disease participants.[159] When people

---

156   Kris Gunnars, "FODMAP 101: A Detailed Beginner's Guide," *Healthline*, November 9, 2018; Susan J. Shepherd et al., "Short-Chain Carbohydrates and Functional Gastrointestinal Disorders," *American Journal of Gastroenterology 108*, no. 5 (April 16, 2013): 707–717.

157   "Understanding FODMAPS," *Canadian Digestive Health Foundation*, accessed January 21, 2021.

158   Rene Wisely, "This Gaseous Culprit Could Be Causing Your Stomach Pain and Constipation," *Michigan Health*, January 8, 2018.

159   Jessica R. Biesiekierski et al., "Gluten Causes Gastrointestinal Symptoms in Subjects Without Celiac Disease: A Double-Blind Randomized Placebo-Controlled Trial," *The American Journal of Gastroenterology 106*, no. 3 (March 2011): 508–14.

started to experience negative side effects from foods containing gluten, Biesiekierski expanded her study to verify if it was the gluten protein that was causing this. While gluten is not a part of the FODMAP group, the two are typically present in the same types of food. When the non-celiac disease participants were switched over to a low-FODMAP diet, no negative side-effects were reported.[160] "We believe non-celiac gluten sensitivity probably does exist, but it's not very common and we have a lot more to do until we fully understand gluten," Biesiekierski stated.[161]

A low-FODMAP diet may serve you better than a gluten-free diet. A low-FODMAP diet may be beneficial to people who suffer from irritable bowel syndrome (IBS), functional gastrointestinal disorders (FGID), and inflammatory bowel disease (IBD) (such as Crohn's disease).[162] Research supports a low-FODMAP diet to be used for first-line therapy in people with IBS, as multiple studies have

---

160 Jessica R. Biesiekierski et al., "No Effects of Gluten in Patients with Self-Reported Non-Celiac Gluten Sensitivity After Dietary Reduction of Fermentable, Poorly Absorbed, Short-Chain Carbohydrates," *Gastroenterology 145*, no. 2 (May 2013): 320-8.e1-3.

161 Eliza Barclay, "Sensitive to Gluten? A Carb in Wheat May Be the Real Culprit," *NPR*, May 22, 2014.

162 Peter R. Gibson and Susan J. Shepherd, "Evidence-Based Dietary Management of Functional Gastrointestinal Symptoms: The FODMAP Approach," *Journal of Gastroenterology and Hepatology 25*, no. 2 (January, 2010); Richard B. Gearry et al., "Reduction of Dietary Poorly Absorbed Short-Chain Carbohydrates (Fodmaps) Improves Abdominal Symptoms in Patients with Inflammatory Bowel Disease-a Pilot Study," *Journal of Crohn's & Colitis 3*, no. 1 (February 2009): 8–14.

shown statistically significant improvement in IBS patients on a FODMAP diet."[163]

In a low-FODMAP diet, you want to avoid foods rich in FODMAPs, which include fruits (such as apples, blackberries, dates, and peaches), sweeteners (such as fructose, HFCS, and honey), dairy (such as cow milk, yogurt, whey protein, and soft cheeses), vegetables (such as asparagus, broccoli, cauliflower, leeks, mushrooms, and peas), legumes (such as beans, chickpeas, and lentils), and wheat (such as bread, pasta, and crackers).[164] If you believe a low FOD-MAP diet may be beneficial to you, please take a deep breath. I know my "foods to avoid" list seems like every food out there; however, it is important to keep in mind this

---

163 Emma P. Halmos et al., "A Diet Low in Fodmaps Reduces Symptoms of Irritable Bowel Syndrome," *Gastroenterology 146*, no. 1 (January 2014): 67–75.e5; H. M. Staudacher et al., "Comparison of Symptom Response Following Advice for a Diet Low in Fermentable Carbohydrates (Fodmaps) Versus Standard Dietary Advice in Patients with Irritable Bowel Syndrome," *Journal of Human Nutrition and Dietetics: The Official Journal of British Dietetic Association 24*, no. 5 (October 2011) 487–95.

164 Kris Gunnars, "FODMAP 101: A Detailed Beginner's Guide," *Healthline*, November 9, 2018; Peter R. Gibson and Susan J Shepherd, "Evidence-Based Dietary Management of Functional Gastrointestinal Symptoms: The FODMAP Approach." *Journal of Gastroenterology and Hepatology 25*, no. 2 (January 2010); Jane G. Muir et al., "Measurement of Short-Chain Carbohydrates in Common Australian Vegetables and Fruits by High-Performance Liquid Chromatography (Hplc)," *Journal of Agricultural and Food Chemistry 57*, no. 2 (January 2009): 554–65; "What Are FODMAPS and What's the Connection to Celiac Disease and Gluten Sensitivity?," *Beyond Celiac*, October 28, 2015.

is a LOW-FODMAP diet, not a FODMAP-free diet. Simply minimizing FODMAPs in your diet should bring beneficial health effects. Do not fear, there is a wide range of low-FODMAP foods you can eat in larger quantities. For starters, not all grains have FODMAPs in them. On this diet, you can still enjoy corn, oats, rice, quinoa, and tapioca.[165] Besides, you do not need to avoid/minimize your consumption of all fruits, sweeteners, dairy products, and vegetables.[166] You can still enjoy fruits like bananas, blueberries, grapefruit, kiwi, oranges, and lemons; sweeteners like maple syrup and stevia; dairy products like hard cheeses; vegetables like peppers, carrots, cucumbers, potatoes, spinach, tomatoes, zucchini, and kale; as well as all fats and oils, most nuts and seeds (except pistachios), most herbs and spices, and a variety of beverages.[167]

If you are going to take one thing from this section, know that although gluten and FODMAPs are found within similar foods, they are not the same. The list of foods on a low-FODMAP diet is not as distinctly definitive as compared to the list

---

165 Kris Gunnars, "FODMAP 101: A Detailed Beginner's Guide," *Healthline*, November 9, 2018.

166 Ibid.

167 Ibid; Peter R. Gibson and Susan J Shepherd, "Evidence-Based Dietary Management of Functional Gastrointestinal Symptoms: The FODMAP Approach." *Journal of Gastroenterology and Hepatology 25*, no. 2 (January, 2010); Jane G. Muir et al., "Measurement of Short-Chain Carbohydrates in Common Australian Vegetables and Fruits by High-Performance Liquid Chromatography (Hplc)," *Journal of Agricultural and Food Chemistry 57*, no. 2 (January 2009): 554–65; "What Are FODMAPS and What's the Connection to Celiac Disease and Gluten Sensitivity?," *Beyond Celiac*, October 28, 2015.

of foods on a gluten-free diet. Please keep in mind that the FODMAP diet is pretty restrictive and could cause nutrient deficiencies if not used carefully. By identifying your discomforts and concerns together with a physician, you can create the perfect diet for you. Everyone may react differently to specific foods, but creating a plan can help ease the transition. Remember that any dramatic dietary shift may cause uncomfortable side effects. Some physicians recommend complete elimination of foods high in FODMAPs at first and then reintroducing them, while others recommend a slower transition. Seeking advice from a qualified professional is always the best option.

NOT ALL GRAINS ARE CREATED EQUAL

Eliminating dietary gluten without a doctor's recommendation can lead to inadequate vitamin, mineral, and fiber consumption. Only a limited number of gluten-free items are enriched to contain the essential vitamins and minerals found within certain gluten products.[168] I want to emphasize that I am saying "certain" instead of all gluten products because "not all grains are created equal."[169] Two main subgroups of grains exist: whole grains and refined grains. Similar to gluten-free foods, refined grains can cause deficiencies in fiber, vitamins, and minerals.

The era of refined grains began in the late 1800s around the time when industrialization skyrocketed in the US. During this time, only whole-grain flour existed; however,

---

168 "Nutrient Deficiencies," *Gluten.org*, accessed January 21, 2021.

169 Stephanie Mitchell et al., "Not All Grains Are Created Equal: Gluten-Free Products Not Included in Mandatory Folate Fortification," *Current Developments in Nutrition* 3, no. 5 (May 2019).

it spoiled easily. The rancidity of wheat flour quickly became a provoking issue. The solution was easy: milling machinery was able to successfully extend the shelf life of flour by removing the bran and the germ, two nutritious parts of the wheat kernel. This was the birth of the well-known all-purpose white flour.[170]

Was the removal of fiber through the milling process really worth the extended shelf life?

Historians, nutritionists, and researchers claim the extended shelf life may not have been worth the consequences of changing the composition of wheat flour. After the emergence of the milling technique, the prevalence of deficiency diseases drastically increased.[171] I acknowledge multiple explanations are possible for this increase of diseases, such as population density, migration, and smoking, but the creation of refined grains plays a major role here as well.

Many people are inclined to buy refined grains such as white flour and white bread because of its finer texture, longer shelf life, and less grainy taste. What many people may not realize is that they are also buying an increased risk of B-vitamin deficiencies (pellagra and beriberi), metabolic syndromes (conditions such as increased blood pressure and high blood sugar that occur together to increase your risk of heart disease, stroke, and type II diabetes), cancers, and more. [172]

170 Catherine Guthrie, "The Truth About Refined Grains," *Experience L!fe*, July 1, 2019.

171 Peter Cox, *You Don't Need Meat* (New York, NY: Thomas Dunne Books, 2002).

172 Mayo Clinic Staff, "Metabolic Syndrome," *Mayo Clinic*, March 14, 2019.

As the negative effects of refined grains became more prominent in society, governments began to require their enrichment. What this means is certain B vitamins (folic acid, niacin, thiamin, riboflavin) and irons were reintroduced to normalize their previously low levels due to the milling technique. Additionally, some refined grains may be fortified, which adds much-needed vitamins and minerals that might not have been there in the first place or at a higher level than what is naturally found.[173] The meticulous observations in human health following the emergence of refined grains allowed for the correction and/or reduction of medical conditions, such as neural tube defects (NTD). The CDC claims the ability to fortify enriched grains has been able to save 1,300 babies each year from suffering from NTD.[174] The association between NTD in babies and folic acid fortification continues to be studied in the Centers for Birth Defects Research and Prevention, which is funded by the CDC.[175] This is just one example of the wonders of using grain fortification.

FIBER:

While most B vitamins and other components of bran and germ can be replenished from enriched and fortified grains, fiber can never be restored. Fiber is an important part of the diet. Numerous studies from the National Cancer Institute

---

173 Juliana Yellin, "Everything You Need to Know About Grains," *Food Insight*, June 27, 2017.

174 "Key Findings: Folic Acid Fortification Continues to Prevent Neural Tube Defect," *Centers for Disease Control and Prevention (CDC)*, last modified November 3, 2017.

175 "Together We Can Discover the Causes of Birth Defects," *National Birth Defects Prevention Study (NBDPS)*, accessed January 22, 2021.

have suggested a 15 and 10 percent reduction of deaths in women and men respectively, with just an increase of 10 grams of fiber in diets.[176] A diet that lacks fiber increases the risks of prostate cancer, appendicitis, digestion issues, and more. [177] Fiber may be the key to restoring your relationship with your gut microbiome. I believe it was a vital factor in helping to clear up my skin.

According to the American Heart Association, it is recommended that American adults on a daily two-thousand-calorie diet consume twenty-five grams of fiber a day.[178] This number may differ slightly, depending upon age and sex. The leading health organizations recommend that children and adults get fourteen grams of fiber for every one thousand calories consumed. This means kids aged four to eight years should receive an estimated twenty-five grams of fiber daily and little ones aged one to three years should receive an estimated nineteen grams of fiber daily.[179] Since the average American consumes fifteen grams of fiber each day, we face the issue of not fulfilling the recommended daily needs.

---

176 "How Proper Fiber Intake Can Change Your Life and Improve Your Diet," *NuGo Fiber*, November 1, 2016; Yikyung Park et al., "Dietary Fiber Intake and Mortality in the NIH-AARP Diet and Health Study," *Archives of Internal Medicine 171*, no. 12 (June 2011): 1061–8.

177 Peter Cox, *You Don't Need Meat* (New York, NY: Thomas Dunne Books, 2002); Larsen, Laura, ed. *Diet and Nutrition Sourcebook* (Detroit, MI: Omnigraphics Inc., 2011); Melina Jampolis, "What Exactly Does Fiber Do," *CNN*, November 8, 2012.

178 "Whole Grains, Refined Grains, and Dietary Fiber," *American Heart Association*, accessed on January 18, 2021.

179 "How Much (Dietary) Fiber Should I Eat?," *USDA*, July 17, 2019; "How Much Fiber Do Children Need?," *Cleveland Clinic*, December 30, 2020.

If the average American were to simply incorporate one ounce of chia seeds a day into their diet, their risk of death could be reduced. This is so easy! Why would we not do this? Refer to the chart below to see other easy ways to increase your fiber intake.

Food Item	Serving Size	Fiber Amount (grams)
Lentils (Boiled)	1 Cup	15.5
Chia Seeds	1 Ounce	10.0
Raspberries	1 Cup	8.0
Broccoli (Boiled)	1 Cup (chopped)	5.0
Quinoa (Cooked)	1 Cup	5.0
Banana	1 Medium	3.0
Whole Wheat Bread	1 Slice	2.0

Table 1: Foods Rich in Fiber. The list of fiber-rich food sources expands well beyond this table, which is designed just to show some examples.[180]

Side note:

One ounce of chia seeds may seem like a lot, but this is equivalent to two tablespoons. A typical chia seed pudding accounts for three to four tablespoons. In my personal experiences with food, I have grown to love chia seeds. The cool thing about chia seeds is that they take on the flavor of whatever they are added to. They are so easy to incorporate into any food. Some examples of what I add chia seeds to are avocado toast, smoothies, salads, and yogurt.

Referring back to our conversation in the Rise of Nutrition chapter about a uniform food label, for food to be

---

180   Mayo Clinic Staff, "Chart of High-Fiber Foods," *Mayo Clinic*, January 5, 2021.

considered a "good source" of fiber it must contain at least three grams per serving, and for a food to be considered an "excellent source" of fiber, it must contain at least five grams per serving.[181] It is important to note that 100 percent natural foods are the best sources of fiber. For example, processed fruit juices do not contain as much fiber as whole fruits.[182]

WHAT IS FIBER?

For the Scientific Reader:

Dietary fibers are non-digestible plant polysaccharides (long-chain carbohydrates), which cause physical barriers between the enzymes in the small intestines. [183] The term "non-digestible" refers to a substance that is not able to be absorbed within the small intestines.[184]

There are two different types of dietary fibers: soluble and insoluble. Soluble dietary fiber turns into a gel-like substance as it dissolves in water, which allows it to slow down digestion by delaying gastric emptying (soluble fiber makes you

---

181 George Ivanoff, *Fiber (What's in My Food?)* (Mankato, MN: Smart Apple Media, 2012).

182 Kerrie K Saunders, *The Vegan Diet as Chronic Disease Prevention* (New York, NY: Lantern Books, 2003).

183 Brian Lindshield, "1.3: Polysaccharides - Fiber," *Medicine LibreTexts*. August 14, 2020; Myriam M.-L Grundy et al., "Re-evaluation of the Mechanisms of Dietary Fibre and Implications for Macronutrient Bioaccessibility, Digestion and Postprandial Metabolism," *The British Journal of Nutrition 116*, no. 5 (July 7, 2016): 816–833.

184 Institute of Medicine , *Dietary Reference Intakes Proposed Definition of Dietary Fiber* (Washington DC: National Academies Press, 2001).

feel fuller for longer).[185] After moving past the small intestines, certain soluble fibers have the potential to break down from bacteria within the large intestines (colon). Insoluble dietary fibers remain intact moving food through the intestines (small and large) more quickly and attracting water to your stool.[186] This is quite astonishing since the digestive tract is twenty-eight feet long.[187] Insoluble dietary fiber is often recommended to treat constipation, as it can lead to softer, bulkier stools that are easier to pass.[188] Keep in mind, your risks of gastrointestinal diseases (such as an ulcer) increase as stool transit time increases.[189] Insoluble fiber has been described to act like a brush, "sweeping through your bowels to get everything out and keep things moving."[190] Fiber is only found within plant products; meat and dairy products do not have fiber. Both types of fiber are found to benefit human health. Interestingly, controversy currently exists regarding the dietary fiber group names. The National Academies of

185 Linda Rath, "Can Increasing Fiber Reduce Inflammation?," *Arthritis Foundation*, accessed January 18, 2021; V. T. Hoang Ho et al., "The Effect of Oat β-Glucan on LDL-Cholesterol, Non-HDL-Cholesterol and ApoB for CVD Risk Reduction: A Systematic Review and Meta-Analysis of Randomised-Controlled Trials," *British Journal of Nutrition 116*, no. 8 (October 11, 2016): 1369–1382.

186 Linda Rath, "Can Increasing Fiber Reduce Inflammation?," *Arthritis Foundation*, accessed

187 January 18, 2021. V. T. Hoang Ho et al., "The Effect of Oat β-Glucan on LDL-Cholesterol, Non-

188 HDL-Cholesterol and ApoB for CVD Risk Reduction: A Systematic Review and Me

189 ta-Analy

190 sis of Randomised-Controlled Trials," *British Journal of Nutrition 116*, no. 8 (October 11, 2016): 1369–1382.

Sciences, Engineering, and Medicine (NASEM) Food and Nutrition Board suggests the categories of soluble and insoluble should be phased out and replaced by viscosity and fermentability.[191] They believe describing the dietary fiber's physicochemical properties may be a more appropriate name.

Refer to the chart below to see some foods that contain dietary soluble and insoluble fibers. It is important to keep in mind that some foods overlap and contain both. If you think a fiber supplement (like Metamucil or Citrucel) may be beneficial to you, ask your doctor.

Soluble Fiber – slows down digestion, full feeling	Insoluble Fiber – easy to pass
Whole grains (such as barley and oatmeal)	Whole grains (such as brown rice and couscous)
Vegetables (such as broccoli, artichokes, and peas)	Root vegetables (such as carrots, potatoes, and onions
Fruits (such as peeled apples, bananas, berries, and oranges)	Fruits with edible seeds (such as berries); fruits with peels (such as apples, peaches, and pears)
Legumes (such as lentils)	Legumes (such as beans and lentils)
Nuts and seeds (such as almonds, flaxseeds, and sesame seeds)	Nuts and seeds

Table 2: Foods that contain soluble and insoluble fibers. This list of soluble and insoluble fiber-rich food sources expands well beyond this table. The table is designed just to show some examples.[192]

---

191 Institute of Medicine, *Dietary Reference Intakes Proposed Definition of Dietary Fiber* (Washington DC: National Academies Press, 2001).

192 "Soluble vs. Insoluble Fiber," *MedlinePlus*, last modified January 5, 2021; "Insoluble Fibre and Diabetes," *Diabetes.co.uk*, January 15, 2019; "Soluble and Insoluble Fiber Food List," *North Ottawa Wellness Foundation*, accessed February 19, 2021.

For the Scientific Reader:

Soluble fiber can aid in lowering low-density lipoprotein (LDL or "bad" cholesterol).[193] We do not want accumulated LDL levels in the bloodstream as it is associated with atherosclerosis and increased risks of cardiovascular disease (CVD). Serum cholesterol is lowered since fiber is non-digestible and, therefore, interferes with the absorption and recycling of cholesterol and bile acids. When fiber travels through the digestive tract, it binds with cholesterol and forces its excretion and prevents the reabsorption into the bloodstream. Dr. Alejandro Junger, a cardiologist, author, and founder of the Clean Program explains that "when we don't eat fiber, the toxins that we should be eliminating through our bowels get reabsorbed into the bloodstream, which can cause many problems."[194] In 2015, research studies showed an 18 percent reduction in cholesterol levels when participants consumed 10 to 25 grams of soluble fiber daily.[195] Ensuring that

193 Linda Rath, "Can Increasing Fiber Reduce Inflammation?," *Arthritis Foundation*, accessed January 18, 2021; V. T. Hoang Ho et al., "The Effect of Oat β-Glucan on LDL-Cholesterol, Non-HDL-Cholesterol and ApoB for CVD Risk Reduction: A Systematic Review and Meta-Analysis of Randomised-Controlled Trials," *British Journal of Nutrition 116*, no. 8 (October 11, 2016): 1369–1382.

194 "Dr. Alejandro Junger," Goop, accessed January 18, 2021; "Fiber: Why It Matters More Than You Think," *Experience L!fe*, accessed on January 18, 2021.

195 Quan Zhou et al., Beneficial Effect of Higher Dietary Fiber Intake on Plasma HDL-C and TC/HDL-C Ratio among Chinese Rural-to-Urban Migrant Workers," *Int. J. Environ. Res. Public Health 12*, no. 5 (April 29, 2015): 4726–4738.

you meet the recommended guidelines of fiber intake may be an important step in reducing your "bad" cholesterol. Specifically, whole grains and vegetables are excellent sources of fiber. The American Heart Association reported that a high-fiber diet can potentially lower cholesterol levels by 10 percent.[196] Insoluble fibers are not shown to have significant roles in adjusting cholesterol levels.

For the Scientific Reader:
Refer back to the conversation on inflammatory biomarkers, such as C-reactive proteins (CRP) within the inflammation chapter. Dr. Dana E. King, professor, and chair of family medicine at West Virginia University in Morgantown, explains why fiber is important in controlling your CRP levels.[197] People who eat high-fiber diets have reported a 25 to 54 percent reduction in CRP blood levels according to a 2009 review in the *European Journal of Clinical Nutrition* publication.[198] So, not only will eating more fiber help your bowel and gut health, it also may be the key to controlling inflammation in your body. As you can see, the human body is very complex.

---

196 "Prevention and Treatment of High Cholesterol," *American Heart Association*, accessed January 18, 2021.

197 Linda Rath, "Can Increasing Fiber Reduce Inflammation?," *Arthritis Foundation*, accessed January 18, 2021.

198 Yunsheng Ma et al., Association Between Dietary Fiber and Serum C-Reactive Protein," *American Journal of Clinical Nutrition 83*, no. 4 (April 2006): 760–766.

Everything is connected back to the gut microbiome. You want to promote the growth of the beneficial microorganisms within your gut microbiome. While most relationships between food and the gut microbiome are less well-known, others are obvious. Prebiotics are fibers that can prompt the growth and activity of the healthy microorganisms in your gut microbiome.[199] Remember how I mentioned that certain soluble fibers may be broken down by bacteria within the large intestines? The types of soluble fibers that are capable of this are the prebiotics, which are also known as fermentable fibers. Bananas, onions, and garlic are foods that naturally contain high levels of prebiotics.[200] Increased quantities of healthy bacteria are the key to maintaining a healthy gut.

IS THERE A LIMIT AS TO HOW MUCH FIBER YOU CAN EAT?

Technically, there is no upper limit established for dietary fiber.[201] While it is rare for an individual to consume an excess of fiber, excess fiber in the body may interfere with digestion and food absorption. To achieve a level of dietary fiber that would be considered hazardous would take a considerable amount of conscious effort. Most likely, dietary sources of fiber would not be sufficient enough to get you to this point, and this issue would arrive as a result of excessive

---

199 Joanne Slavin, "Fiber and Prebiotics: Mechanisms and Health Benefits," *Nutrients 5*, no. 4 (April 2013): 1417–35.

200 Arlene Semeco, "The 19 Best Prebiotic Foods You Should Eat," *Healthline*, June 8, 2016.

201 Paula Trumbo et al., "Dietary Reference Intakes for Energy, Carbohydrate, Fiber, Fat, Fatty Acids, Cholesterol, Protein and Amino Acids," *Journal of the American Dietetic Association 102*, no. 11 (November 2002): 1621–1630.

supplementation. It is always a good idea to get your fiber sources naturally from food.

Before you change your diet to include foods high in fiber, it is important to note that you must increase your fiber levels gradually. Any drastic change in diet will take your body time to adjust. It is recommended to make small weekly diet changes, such as adding an additional serving of fruits or vegetables to your diet. Remember "you are what you eat," and if you were previously relaxed about the levels of fiber within your diet, the microorganisms in your gut microbiome are not accustomed to breaking down fiber. Raising your fiber intake gradually each day will yield positive outcomes for your body and gut microbiome.

When your body is not used to digesting certain substances, it can produce unwanted effects such as bloating, abdominal pain, and constipation. To alleviate some of this discomfort, try increasing your water intake.[202] Water helps fiber travel through the digestive system. Dr. Jacqueline Wolf, a gastroenterologist and associate professor of medicine at Harvard Medical School, recommends drinking eight or nine glasses of water every day.[203]

THE GRAIN KERNEL:

While enriched grains are a way to restore the damage created by refined grains, it still does not make them nutritionally equal to whole grains. As previously stated, "not all grains are created equal," and whole grains are the superior

---

202 Natalie Butler, "Can You Actually Ingest Too Much Fiber?," *Healthline*, April 16, 2019.

203 "Rethinking Fiber and Hydration Can Lead to Better Colon Health," *Harvard Health*, August 2013.

choice. This is because whole grains include the entire grain kernel with the bran, germ, and endosperm.

THE BRAN

The outer layer of the wheat kernel is referred to as the bran, and it contains fiber, B vitamins, and antioxidants. In the body, a balance exists between free radicals and antioxidants for adequate physiological function. Free radicals may damage cells and interfere with critical homeostatic mechanisms by attacking macromolecules in the body.[204] Antioxidants have the power to slow down this damage. An example of an antioxidant in whole grains are phytochemicals, which are found naturally in plant-based foods. Phytochemicals are considered to be anti-inflammatories.[205]

THE GERM

The germ makes up the core of the wheat kernel. A wheat germ is in charge of reproducing a new wheat sprout. This good germ is an excellent source of nutrients, explaining why it is so detrimental when removed from refined grains. The germ provides healthy fats, B vitamins (like thiamin-B1 and folate-B9), minerals (like magnesium, phosphorus, and zinc), and even a source of protein.[206] Interestingly, you can buy and eat the wheat germ alone. It is available in its raw form and is commonly used as a topping for yogurts and

---

204 V. Lobo et al., "Free Radical, Antioxidants and Functional Foods: Impact on Human Health," *Pharmacognosy Reviews* 4, no. 8 (Jul-Dec 2010): 118–26.

205 Natalie Olsen, "Phytonutrients," *Healthline*, May 25, 2019.

206 "Health Foods," *Mayo Clinic*, April 5, 2019.

ice cream. Try substituting breadcrumbs for wheat germ![207] Bob's Red Mill makes an excellent wheat germ that has a nutty and toasted flavor.[208] Finally, a germ that is thought of in a positive way.

THE ENDOSPERM

The largest part of the wheat kernel is the endosperm, accounting for the middle layer. The endosperm is the only region of the kernel that remains in refined grains. Although the endosperm plays a critical role in providing essential energy and support for embryonic growth (since it is mostly composed of starches with some vitamins and proteins), 25 percent of protein concentration in grains are lost without the other two layers of the kernel: the bran and the germ.[209]

WHAT FOODS CAN I FIND WHOLE GRAINS IN AND HOW MUCH SHOULD I EAT?

It is not always easy to distinguish between whole, refined, and enriched grains. People are often misguided to believe all brown breads are whole wheat. The brown coloring may not always be natural—it may come from additives.[210] Additionally, just because bread has the words "whole wheat" on the packaging does not mean that it is a true whole

207 Natalie Olsen, "How Wheat Germ Benefits Your Health," *Healthline*, September 17, 2018.

208 "What Is Wheat Germ and Why Should I Be Eating It?," *Bob's Red Mill*, January 31, 2019.

209 "What Is a Whole Grain," *Oldways Whole Grains Council*, accessed January 22, 2021.

210 "Whole Gains vs. Regular Grains: What's the Difference?," *The Mayo Clinic Diet*, accessed January 22, 2021.

grain. According to the FDA, "the ingredients are listed in order of predominance, with the ingredients used in the greatest amount first, followed in descending order by those in smaller amounts."[211] When looking at the nutrition label, if you find the words "unbleached enriched flour" before "whole wheat flour," then this is not a true whole grain bread. According to the Mayo Clinic, when searching for whole grain bread, for example, a key trick is to look for the first ingredient to start with the word "whole" or make sure that the packaging says "100 percent whole grain."[212] One-hundred percent whole grain items should contain sixteen grams of whole grains.[213] The Mayo Clinic also recommends trying white whole wheat bread if you want the nutritional benefits of whole wheat but prefer the taste and texture of white bread.[214] Surprisingly, white whole wheat bread is made completely of whole grains (it contains all three parts of the kernel). White whole-wheat bread has a softer texture and milder flavor compared to brown whole-wheat bread. The difference in colors is because white wheat lacks the bran coloring, while red wheat used in whole-wheat bread is much darker and has a coarser texture. There are no negative consequences to choosing white whole wheat bread, just make

211 "Overview of Food Ingredients, Additives & Colors," *FDA*, last modified February 6, 2018.

212 Katherine Zeratsky, "How Can Bread Be Labeled as Both White and Whole Wheat? Is White Whole-Wheat Bread a Healthy Choice?," *Mayo Clinic*, January 18, 2020.

213 "2015-2020 Dietary Guidelines," *Health.gov*, accessed January 22, 2021.

214 Katherine Zeratsky, "How Can Bread Be Labeled as Both White and Whole Wheat? Is White Whole-Wheat Bread a Healthy Choice?," *Mayo Clinic*, January 18, 2020.

sure to use the nutrition and ingredient labels to properly identify your whole grains.

The United States Department of Agriculture (USDA) recommends that whole grains constitute half of your daily grain consumption.[215] The amount of whole grains you should eat varies for each individual depending on your age, sex, and activity level.[216] If you are following a two-thousand-calorie daily diet, the Dietary Guidelines for Americans advise you to consume six one-ounce grain servings a day.[217] To translate this, one slice of bread or half a cup of cooked pasta would equal a one-ounce serving of grains.

A majority of Americans consume the recommended levels of grains; however, only a few of these grains are whole grains.[218] Registered dietitian and nutritionist Megan Holdaway shares tips on how to incorporate whole grains into meals. There are over twenty different types of whole grains, some of which may be new to you. Everyone is familiar with the typical whole wheat bread, oats, and quinoa, but have you ever heard of einkorn, spelt, or teff?[219]

Holdaway recommends narrowing your options. Before you go exploring the variety of whole grains, choose just

215 Lisa Mancino and Jean C. Buzby, "Americans' Whole-Grain Consumption Below Guidelines," *Economic Research Service: United States Department of Agriculture*, April 1, 2005.

216 "What Foods are in the Grains Group?," *MyPlate: U.S. Department of Agriculture*, accessed January 22, 2021.

217 "2015–2020 Dietary Guidelines," *Health.gov*, accessed January 22, 2021.

218 Juliana Yellin, "Everything You Need to Know About Grains," *Food Insight*, June 27, 2017.

219 "Whole Grains A to Z," *Oldways Whole Grains Council*, accessed January 22, 2021.

two whole grains and learn how to prepare them in ways palatable for you. One example of this may be as simple as replacing cereal with oatmeal or replacing your refined white flour with a whole wheat version.[220] Personally, I like the nutty flavor of whole wheat pasta; however, if you dislike this taste, then try switching out a different refined grain for whole grain. Similar to other foods, pasta can be prepared in numerous ways. The chosen cooking method can alter the nutrient contents as explained with high-temperature cooking in red meats. If you do not choose to eat whole wheat pasta, it is recommended to cook your pasta al dente; it lowers the glycemic index.

For the Scientific Reader:

The glycemic index ranks food on a scale from zero to one-hundred based on how much your blood sugar will rise because of it. A lower ranking indicates a slower rise. The glycemic index does not indicate the upper limit of your blood sugar after you eat a specific food.[221] The glycemic load measure can indicate this, so make sure you research both the glycemic index and load if you choose to further investigate this concept. Al dente penne pasta reported a glycemic index of fifty.[222] To put this into perspective, Harvard

---

220 "Grains," *Let's Eat Healthy*, accessed January 22, 2021.

221 "The Lowdown on Glycemic Index and Glycemic Load," *Harvard Health*, last modified April 10, 2020.

222 F Scaazzina et al., "Glycemic Index and Glycemic Load of Commercial Italian Foods," *Nutrition, Metabolism, and Cardiovascular Diseases (NMCD)* 25, no. 5 (February 2016): 419–29.

Health presented the glycemic index of rolled oats to be fifty-five.[223]

WHAT IF YOU MUST FOLLOW A GLUTEN-FREE DIET?

People often assume all grains contain gluten; however, this is not the case. There are plenty of naturally gluten-free grains, such as rice, quinoa, buckwheat, flax, and millet. Once again, it is always recommended to read the nutrition labels, since each food item may differ based on the brand.

For an item to be considered "gluten-free," it must have less than twenty parts per million of gluten according to the US FDA guidelines.[224] For example, many alcoholic beverages that contain gluten may have undergone processing to remove the gluten; this can be identified in a label that states "processed," "treated," or "crafted" to remove gluten. Due to the FDA rules, these beers are still not able to say gluten-free because they are unable to determine their exact gluten content. As a result, the labels must explain that "the beverage may contain some gluten."[225]

The protein gluten is found in all wheat (including durum, einkorn, emmer, kamut, and spelt), barley, rye, and triticale.[226] Therefore, if you are gluten-free, you want to avoid these food ingredients. As previously mentioned, a gluten-free diet will change your intake of nutrients. While whole grains may

223 "Glycemic Index for 60+ Foods," *Harvard Health*, last modified January 6, 2020.

224 "'Gluten-Free' Means What It Says," *FDA*, last modified January 11, 2021.

225 Mayo Clinic Staff, "Gluten-Free Diet," *Mayo Clinic*, December 19, 2019.

226 Megan Ware, "Everything You Need to Know About Gluten," *Medical-NewsToday*, July 17, 2018.

provide an excellent source of fiber and B-vitamins they are not the only source.

B VITAMINS

All B vitamins play a role in converting foods into energy. B vitamins can be found in grains, meats, eggs, dairy, legumes, vegetables, fruits, nuts, and seeds. There are eight different types of B vitamins: thiamin (B1), riboflavin (B2), niacin (B3), pantothenic acid (B5), pyridoxine (B6), biotin (B7), Folate (B9), and cyanocobalamin (B12).[227] Also, all B vitamins are water-soluble, meaning that the body is not able to store them, and, after usage, the body can excrete them. It is essential to replenish your B vitamins daily. Although B vitamins are found in many foods, they are easily denatured if prepared the wrong way. It is especially important to watch out for the triggers of B vitamin destruction when gluten is removed from the diet. Here are three popular examples:

RIBOFLAVIN (B2)

Riboflavin (B2) plays an important role in energy production within the body.[228] Fortunately, deficiencies in riboflavin are atypical, but they are possible. Chances of experiencing ariboflavinosis (B2 deficiency) are elevated with chronic alcohol abuse, since it may prevent your body from absorbing other nutrients, and with people who do not consume dairy, since a large source of riboflavin comes from milk-based products.[229]

---

227 "Vitamin B," *Better Health*, last modified May 2020.

228 Hector D'Souza, "Vitamin B2," *NDHealth* Facts, last modified March 17, 2014.

229 "Vitamin B," *Better Health*, last modified May 2020.

Think back to the last time you went food shopping and bought a carton of milk. There are many fat percentages and brands available. On top of that, have you ever noticed the physical presentation of these milks? Some of them are typically found in smaller cartons, such as Horizon and Stonyfield, while others can be found in the large gallon jugs (most people tend to think of these as the store brand).

Look past the major differences in these presentations. What is the same? Think about the different options of buying orange juice at the grocery store. You have similar colored cartons, but you also have the clear bottles. Have you ever wondered why it is unusual to find milk in a clear bottle or why milk is always stored in opaque containers? Unlike the previous cooking techniques that alter nutrient absorption in red meats, riboflavin is denatured by light. Milk that is stored in clear bottles loses 50 percent of its riboflavin after only two hours of exposure to bright light, so milk is kept in opaque containers to avoid light degradation. [230]

Unfortunately, not all milk brands follow this unspoken rule. Milk found in clear bottles may be tempting to buy, because the clear glass bottle stands out and looks good on the shelves; however, the chances that this milk has been on the shelves for more than two hours are high. As a result, the percentages of riboflavin are low within these milks.

PANTOTHENIC ACID (B5)

All eight of the B vitamins are responsible for aiding in the conversion of the three macronutrients (fats, carbohydrates,

---

230 H. Böhles, "Antioxidative Vitamins in Prematurely and Maturely Born Infants," *International Journal for Vitamin and Nutrition Research 67*, no. 5 (1997): 321–8.

and protein) into energy. Panthothenic acid (B5) stands out for creating blood cells and hormones related to stress and sex. Panthothenic acid is necessary to synthesize cholesterol and can be found in nearly everything. [231] This comes as no surprise, since the Greek word *pantou* literally translates to "everywhere."[232]

The bioavailability of pantothenic acid averages to around 50 percent.[233] The measure of bioavailability is able to tell us the proportion of which nutrient is digested, absorbed, and metabolized.[234] This means that only 50 percent of pantothenic acid actually reaches the systemic circulation.[235] Similar to red meats, high-temperature cooking creates negative health outcomes. In this case, extensive high-temperature cooking along with the processes of canning, freezing, and refining, destroy some pantothenic acid, therefore lowering the bioavailability. When in doubt, try to eat fresh foods.

---

231 "Vitamin B5 (Pantothenic Acid)," *Mount Sinai*, accessed January 22, 2021.

232 Piriya Mahendra Pordes, "Vitamin B5 (Pantothenic Acid): Benefits, Best Sources, Dosage, Deficiency," *Netdoctor*, March 6, 2020.

233 National Institutes of Health, *The National Academies: Dietary Reference Intakes for Thiamin, Riboflavin, Niacin, Vitamin B6, Folate, Vitamin B12, Pantothenic Acid, Biotin and Choline* (Washington DC: National Academies Press, 1998).

234 V. Srini Srinivasan, "Bioavailability of Nutrients: A Practical Approach to in Vitro Demonstration of the Availability of Nutrients in Multivitamin-Mineral Combination Products," *The Journal of Nutrition 131*, no. 4 (April 2001): 1349S–1350S.

235 Clive Cannons et al., "What is Bioavailability and Bioequivalence?," *Best Practice (Journal)* (July, 2009): 4–8.

BIOTIN (B7)

Biotin (B7), also known as vitamin H, plays an important role in gene regulation, genome stability, and other cellular processes.[236] Biotin contributes to converting food into energy and maintaining healthy skin, hair, eyes, liver, and the nervous system.[237]

It is likely that you are fulfilling the recommended amount of biotin from the foods you eat, in addition to the fact that our bodies can release free biotin from the bacteria in our large intestines.[238] However, if you are looking to increase your biotin levels naturally apart from whole grains, great sources of biotin can be found in meats, poultry, dairy products, eggs, certain legumes (peas, beans, lentils), nuts, and vegetables such as cabbage, broccoli, potatoes, and mushrooms.[239]

---

236 Mahendra P. Singh et al., "Biotinylation of Lysine 16 in Histone H4 Contributes Toward Nucleosome Condensation," *Archives of Biochemistry and Biophysics 529*, no. 2 (January 2013): 105–11; Toshinobu Kuroishi et al., "Biotinylation Is a Natural, Albeit Rare, Modification of Human Histones," *Molecular Genetics and Metabolism 104*, no. 4 (December 2011): 537–45; National Institutes of Health, *The National Academies: Dietary Reference Intakes for Thiamin, Riboflavin, Niacin, Vitamin B6, Folate, Vitamin B12, Pantothenic Acid, Biotin and Choline* (Washington DC: National Academies Press, 1998).

237 Cara J Stevens, "Health Benefits of Biotin," *Healthline*, March 8, 2019.

238 O. M. Wrong et al., "The Large Intestine: Its Role in Mammalian Nutrition and Homeostasis," *Quarterly Journal of Experimental Physiology 67*, no. 2 (April 1982): 217.

239 Rebecca Morris, "What Does Vitamin B5 Do?," *Healthline*, last modified August 15, 2018.

It is important to note that the positives of biotin in eggs are found only in cooked eggs. To some people, this point of clarification is obvious; although there are people that imitate Sylvester Stallone's notorious movie character Rocky, a Philadelphian boxing legend, and consume raw eggs as a quick way to increase their protein intake. People regularly consume raw egg whites when sneaking a piece of raw cookie dough or a spoonful of cake batter. Not only do medical professionals advise against the consumption of raw eggs (due to salmonella), they warn that raw egg whites contain a protein called avidin that could potentially cause negative health effects as it binds to biotin, preventing its absorption.[240]

For the Scientific Reader

You may recall the words "avidin" or "biotin" from chemistry or biology laboratories. In high-affinity protein-ligand interactions, the avidin-biotin complex is a model system as it is the strongest investigated non-covalent interaction (equilibrium dissociation constant = 10–15M). This complex is resilient to changes in the pH, temperature, and additional denaturing agents.[241]

240 Carol Byrd-Bredbenner et al., *Wadlwar's Perspectives in Nutrition Ninth Edition* (New York: McGraw-Hill Education, 2012); Ellie Whitney and Sharon Rady Rolfes, *Understanding Nutrition Eleventh Edition* (Belmont, California: Wadsworth Publishing Company, 2008).

241 T. Sano et al., "Genetic Engineering of Streptavidin, a Versatile Affinity Tag," *Journal of Chromatography 715*, no. 1 (1998): 85–91; P S Stayton et al., "Streptavidin-Biotin Binding Energetics," *Biomolecular Engineering 16*, no. 1-4 (December 1999): 39–44; O H Laitinen et al., "Genetically Engineered Avidins and Streptavidins," *Cellular and Molecular Life Sciences 63*, no. 24 (December 2006): 2992–3017.

Scientists use the avidin-biotin complex as a secondary antibody to detect and collect specific primary target reagents, such as antibodies and ligands to study.[242] The avidin-biotin complex is used in laboratory settings under the experiments of western, northern, and southern blotting, immunoprecipitation, cell surface labeling, fluorescence-activated cell sorting (FACS), electrophoretic mobility shift assay (EMSA), immunohistochemistry (IHC), and enzyme-linked immunosorbent assay (ELISA). These applications allow for the research and investigation on protein isolation and identification, antibody and protein measurements, cell purification, and more.[243]

THE POWERS OF WHEATGRASS

It is important to know whether or not you tolerate gluten. A plant called *Triticum Aestivum* is responsible for the creation of the superfood wheatgrass. Food can only be classified as a superfood if it contains a rich source of antioxidants, fiber, fatty acids, and other compounds, and promotes human

242 "Avidin-Biotin Interaction," *ThermoFisher Scientific*, accessed January 22, 2021.

243 Ibid; Xiaofeng Liao et al., "Fluorescence-Activated Cell Sorting for Purification of Plasmacytoid Dendritic Cells from the Mouse Bone Marrow," *Journal of Visualized Experiments 117*, (November 2016): 54641; Claire Horlock, "Enzyme-Linked Immunosorbent Assay (ELISA)," *British Society for Immunology, Imperial College London*, accessed January 22, 2021.

health benefits.[244] Wheatgrass contains anti-inflammatory, antioxidant, and antibacterial characteristics due to the extensive combination of nutrients to enhance overall health.[245]

Flour is made by grinding together the seeds of grass, and when the grain is exposed to oxygen, we destroy some of the nutrients within it. Grains can be sprouted instead! Sprouted grains activate enzymes to increase metabolism and allow for easier digestion through a better conversion of starches to simple sugars. Similarly, the degradation of storage proteins from the sprouting process increases the bioavailability of these foods.[246] If you have ever heard of Ezekiel bread, they are created through the sprouting process, which explains why Ezekiel bread contains a richer source of fiber and other nutrients compared to other bread types.[247]

Wheatgrass is a complete protein and includes fully available nutrients and antioxidants at high concentration since it is created from the sprouting process of grains.[248] The elevated quantities of enzymes in wheatgrass aid in the body's digestion process, which can lead to the well-known

244 *Merriam-Webster*, s.v. "Superfood (n.)," accessed February 19, 2021; "What Makes Superfood So Super?," *UCDavis*, accessed January 24, 2021.

245 Emily Cronkleton, "Wheatgrass Benefits: 11 Reasons to Enjoy," *Health-line*, last modified on October 12, 2017.

246 Paolo Beninicasa et al., "Sprouted Grains: A Comprehensive Review," *Nutrients 11*, no. 2 (February 2019): 421.

247 Kris Gunnars, "Why Ezekiel Bread Is the Healthiest Bread You Can Eat," *Healthline*, May 22, 2018.

248 Paolo Beninicasa et al., "Sprouted Grains: A Comprehensive Review," *Nutrients 11*, no. 2 (February 2019): 421.

"detox effects" of wheatgrass.[249] Many people associate wheatgrass with the wheatgrass shots you can get at a juicer for this sole purpose.

The aid in digestion may also alleviate uncomfortable digestion symptoms, such as constipation, excess gas, bloating, and other digestive pains.[250] Wheatgrass is thought to eliminate toxins from the body through its abundance and variety of nutrients. For example, chlorophyll makes up 70 percent of wheatgrass and is comparable to hemoglobin in the blood, which is why wheatgrass is sometimes referred to as "green blood."[251] Chlorophyll is able to detoxify the liver and guard the body against carcinogens, substances that have the potential to lead to cancer.[252] Both wheatgrass and chlorophyll are examples of phytonutrients, a natural chemical produced by plants that work to not only eliminate toxins but to strengthen the immune system by creating a resistance to diseases.[253] Also, the nutrient-density of wheatgrass allows you to feel fuller longer, which will reduce your

---

249   Satyavati Rana et al., "Living Life the Natural Way- Wheatgrass and Health," *Functional Foods in Health and Disease 11*, (November 2011): 444–456.

250   Gil Bar-Sela et al., "The Medical Use of Wheatgrass: Review of the Gap Between Basic and Clinical Applications," *Mini Reviews in Medicinal Chemistry 15*, no. 12 (2015): 1002–10.

251   Pawar Kiran Bhikaji et al., "The Effect of Wheatgrass Juice on Hemoglobin Level W.S.R to Samanya-Vishesha Siddhanta," *International Journal of Ayurveda and Pharma Research 3*, no. 7 (July 2015).

252   Satyavati Rana et al., "Living Life the Natural Way- Wheatgrass and Health," *Functional Foods in Health and Disease 11*, (November 2011): 444–456.

253   Ibid.

cravings and has the potential to aid in weight loss and boost your metabolism.[254]

When I first began to investigate the benefits of wheatgrass, I became really invested in reading the experiences and perspectives of other people on the subject. I stumbled across the personal healthy journey of Dr. Eric Berg, a chiropractor and health educator.

Growing up with various injuries, a lot of stress, not a lot of sleep, and blood sugar issues, Dr. Berg realized he had to make a switch from the unhealthy grains and sugars that made up his diet to a diet rich in vegetables and proteins.[255] As Dr. Berg became more educated on the science of nutrition and how food could heal, he became more aware of how the food he ate was changing the composition of his gut microbiome, biologically. One time after a full day of eating pasta, pizza, and cakes, Dr. Berg experienced uncomfortable symptoms while trying to fall asleep, such as a pulse-pounding in his ear. Immediately, Dr. Berg was able to recognize the refined grains in his body were forcing his heart to work harder and led to a slight potassium deficiency. Dr. Berg was motivated to live a healthier life starting with the food on his plate.

Dr. Berg quit his full-time chiropractor job and started teaching and writing "to help people understand health in a simple way."[256] In his clinic, he investigated which nutrient-dense foods could heal people faster and ended up

254 Gil Bar-Sela et al., "The Medical Use of Wheatgrass: Review of the Gap Between Basic and Clinical Applications," *Mini Reviews in Medicinal Chemistry* 15, no. 12 (2015): 1002–10.

255 Eric Berg, "Dr. Berg's Story," *DrBerg*, accessed January 24, 2021.

256 Ibid.

researching wheatgrass. He founded a company that grew wheatgrass over ancient salt beds in Utah, which permitted the wheatgrass the ability to intake seventy-four trace minerals from the earth. The staff at Dr. Berg's clinic, including Dr. Berg himself, began to consume this wheatgrass and reported back nothing but positive remarks.

"It is like drinking liquid sunshine"

- DR. ERIC BERG[257]

In my personal experiences with wheatgrass, I would disagree with the quote above regarding the taste. Before having my first glass of wheatgrass, I expected the taste to be strong, and that is why I decided to blend it with a banana smoothie. I drink banana smoothies as a treat; however, the wheatgrass taste was so strong, it was ruining one of my favorite treats. I knew that I needed to find a different mixture to consume the wheatgrass. After some time experimenting, I found that if you blend the wheatgrass with ice, orange juice, and water, the wheatgrass becomes extremely diluted and the taste is lost to the oranges. Believe me, this is a good thing. Do not give up if you dislike the taste at first. Experiment with different recipes.

In a conversation with Dr. Lauren Rosen, an internal medicine specialist, she emphasized the importance of understanding that wheatgrass supplement pills and powders are not FDA approved. There is no FDA oversight of

---

257 *Eric Berg*, "Wheat- Health Destroyer or Body Healer?," December 31, 2012, video, 8:28.

supplements. I will go into further detail on this in the Supplements chapter.

> "There is no one who is looking in the bottle that you are getting and making sure that it is safe and does not contain harmful toxins."
>
> – DR. ROSEN

I believe in the power of wheatgrass, but if you are taking it in any form less than what is naturally found from the earth, please consult a doctor to ensure how valid it is. If fresh wheatgrass is not available for you to purchase, try making your own wheatgrass. It is super easy!

- Soak two cups of wheatgrass seeds overnight.
- Compact coconut coir to the bottom of a tray, and evenly cover the wheatgrass seeds on top.
- Cover the tray with a paper towel.
- Pour water over the paper towel, which will soak the coconut coir.
- Place this near a window.
- When the paper towel starts to dry up within two days, rewater the paper towel so the wheat seeds to get a source of water.
  - Poke the coconut coir to see if it is dried out. If so, water.
- Around day nine, the wheatgrass will be ready to be juiced!

When your body is given the proper nutrients and nutrient-dense food, you will start to crave those types of foods. Hence, the birth of the well-known saying, "you are what you eat."

You can enjoy wheatgrass regardless of whether or not you can tolerate gluten, because wheatgrass does not contain any gluten. This may come as a surprise to some. Remember that not all grains contain gluten. Gluten is only found within the seed kernels of wheat plants, and since wheatgrass is actually a grass, it does not contain gluten. While risks exist of cross-contamination, it is always smart to check the nutrition labels of different brands of wheatgrass for gluten (if this applies to you).[258] If you have celiac disease, it might be a good idea for a doctor to recommend the brand and type of wheatgrass for you to explore. If you do not follow a gluten-free diet, you may also want to consult a physician, especially if you are on blood-thinning medication, because wheatgrass is high in vitamin K (a blood-clotting agent).[259]

Everywhere you look, people are going gluten-free. Be sure to discuss your diet with your doctor before you hop on the bandwagon and reach for the "GF" products in the supermarkets.

---

258 "Is Wheatgrass Gluten-Free?," *Beyond Celiac*, accessed January 24, 2021.

259 Satyavati Rana et al., "Living Life the Natural Way- Wheatgrass and Health," *Functional Foods in Health and Disease 11*, (November 2011): 444–456.

FIVE

FATS

—

Better Than Expected

I want you to close your eyes and envision the first thing that comes to your mind when you hear the word "fat." I am willing to place bets that the majority of you are envisioning a person who is overweight and some of you may feel uncomfortable with this word. In 2016, WatchCut, a media/news company, conducted a study and created a video to spread awareness of the word association of "fat" in people who have previously struggled with an eating disorder.[260] While some embraced it, the overall consensus agreed that "fat" is an uncomfortable word. I understand the most common meaning of the word "fat" is used in a negative connotation toward an overweight individual; however, the beauty of surviving the struggle of an eating disorder is seeing the power of food. Out of the fifteen individuals asked, only one woman responded to the word "fat" by discussing the health

---

260 *Cut*, "Fat| Eating Disorders| One Word| Cut," February 22, 2016, video, 2:42.

benefits of certain fats on your body and in your food.[261] The word "fat" has over ten different meanings, yet one of the last meanings of the word to come to mind is my favorite one: dietary fat. Unfortunately, societal norms have placed a stigma and a narrowed vision when using the word "fat." Will there ever be a day when dietary fat is the first fat to come to mind?

This chapter goes into science much more than the other chapters in this book. Fats are a very complicated subject, but they are extremely important to understand. I use a lot of terminology. Some terms are lengthy, so I use acronyms after initially introducing the word. To help keep track of all of the acronyms used, please refer to this chart, as needed.

Acronym	Word	Acronym	Word
ALA	Alpha-Lino-lenic	DHA	Docosahexae-noic Acid
BHB	Beta-Hy-droxybutyrate	HDL (healthy=-good)	High-Density Lipoprotein
EPA	Eicosapentae-noic Acid	LDL (lousy=bad)	Low-Density Lipoprotein
CVD	Cardiovascu-lar Disease	Linoleic Acid	Linoleic Acid
AA	Arachidonic Acid	D5D	Delta-5-De-saturase
D6D	Delta-6-De-saturase		

Table 1: Frequently used acronyms mentioned in this chapter.

---

261 Ibid.

Unfortunately, fat, even in dietary terms, is typically associated with a negative connotation. However, in this chapter, I am going to share how fat can be beneficial in our diet by explaining the different types of fat: polyunsaturated, monounsaturated, saturated, and trans fats.[262]

For the Scientific Reader:

Fat molecules are made up of a glycerol backbone (organic molecules with hydrogen and oxygen groups and a fatty acid tail (long hydrogen and carbon chains attached to a carboxyl group).[263]

Cholesterol is another type of fat found in your blood. Understanding cholesterol is critical in distinguishing between the four major types of dietary fat.

For the Scientific Reader:

Cholesterol plays a major role in cell membrane fluidity, which is significant for the structure, function, and signaling of proteins and enzymes. Hormones such as estrogen and testosterone are able to be recruited from cholesterol.[264] While cholesterol is found within the blood, it cannot travel alone through the bloodstream. It requires proteins. When cholesterol and proteins biochemically assemble for transportation,

262 "Dietary Fats," *American Heart Association*, accessed January 27, 2021.

263 "Lipids," *Khan Academy*, accessed January 27, 2021.

264 "Cell Membrane Fluidity," *Khan Academy*, accessed February 15, 2021.

they are referred to as lipoproteins (lipid is another name for fat).

Many different types of cholesterol exist, and the wrong ratio/levels can be detrimental. The two main types are low-density lipoprotein (LDL) ("bad" cholesterol) and high-density lipoprotein (HDL) ("good" cholesterol).

WHAT MAKES LDL BAD?

As LDL cholesterol is carried from the liver to the bloodstream, it can over-accumulate and cling to the arterial wall. This process is called atherosclerosis. Over time, if atherosclerosis continues, blood flow will become restricted. At the same time, blood clots can then cause a clog in the artery, which can ultimately lead to heart disease, strokes, peripheral artery disease (PAD), and/or other cardiovascular diseases (CVD).[265]

WHAT MAKES HDL GOOD?

On the other hand, HDL cholesterol can work to clear the blood of LDL cholesterol. HDL cholesterol can transport LDL cholesterol from the arteries and back toward the liver, which allows the LDL cholesterol to break down and eventually be eliminated from the body.[266] Due to this action, low levels of HDL cholesterol are associated with a higher risk of heart disease.

To help remember which is the good and which is the bad type, think of the "L" in LDL cholesterol as "lousy" and

265 "HDL (Good), LDL (Bad) Cholesterol and Triglycerides," *American Heart Association*, last modified November 6, 2020.

266 Ibid.

the "H" in HDL cholesterol as "healthy."[267] Similar to how there are "good" and "bad" cholesterols, there are "good" and "bad" fats. Unsaturated fats are commonly referred to as the "good" fats and saturated fats are commonly referred to as the "bad" fats.

For the Scientific Reader:

Chemically speaking, in unsaturated fatty acids, some of the hydrogen bonds have been replaced with double bonds between carbon atoms. While monounsaturated fats contain only one double bond, polyunsaturated fats contain at least two (mono means one and poly means many).

A fatty acid has two long hydrocarbon chains. Saturated fatty acids are chains that are flexible which allows them to pack together tightly. Unsaturated fatty acids have double bonds that add structural rigidity and prevent the fatty acids from packing together tightly. This tightness and packing can explain why butter, a saturated fat, is solid while olive oil, a monounsaturated fat, is liquid at room temperature.

MONOUNSATURATED FATS

Unsaturated fats are divided into monounsaturated and polyunsaturated fats. Great sources of monounsaturated fats can be found in avocados, olives (and olive oil), and most tree nuts (e.g., almond, cashew, hazelnuts, peanuts, pistachios,

---

267 Mary L. Gavin, "What's Cholesterol?," *Kids Health*, September 2018.

and others).[268] Diets high in monounsaturated fats show evidence for reducing heart disease risks because they increase HDL cholesterol.[269] Monounsaturated fats may additionally be able to reduce LDL cholesterol directly.[270]

People who follow a Mediterranean diet, which is largely made up of monounsaturated fats, have reported significantly less inflammatory biomarkers, such as C-reactive proteins (CRPs) and interleukin-6 (IL-6) in the body (refer to the Inflammation chapter if you want a refresher on inflammatory biomarkers) Increasing the levels of healthy fats, specifically monounsaturated fats, may be the key to decreasing mortality and ultimately living a healthy life with less inflammation.[271]

---

268 Katherine Zeratsky, What Are MUFAs, and Should I Include Them in My Diet?," *Mayo Clinic*, April 28, 2020.

269 A. Garg, "High-Monounsaturated-Fat Diets for Patients with Diabetes Mellitus: A Meta-Analysis," *The American Journal of Clinical Nutrition* 67, no. 3 (1998): 577S–582S.

270 C. M. Williams et al., "Cholesterol Reduction Using Manufactured Foods High in Monounsaturated Fatty Acids: A Randomized Crossover Study," *The British Journal of Nutrition 81*, no. 6 (June 1999): 439–446.

271 M. de Lorgeril et al., "Mediterranean Diet, Traditional Risk Factors, and the Rate of Cardiovascular Complications After Myocardial Infarction: Final Report of the Lyon Diet Heart Study," *Circulation 99*, no. 6 (February 1999): 779–785; Katherine Esposito et al., "Effect of a Mediterranean-Style Diet on Endothelial Dysfunction and Markers of Vascular Inflammation in the Metabolic Syndrome: A Randomized Trial," *JAMA 292*, no. 12 (September 2004): 1440–1446; Christina Chrysohoou et al., "Adherence to the Mediterranean Diet Attenuates Inflammation and Coagulation Process in Healthy Adults: The ATTICA Study," *Journal of the American College of Cardiology 44*, no. 1 (July 2004): 152–158.

Olive oil is the most common monounsaturated fat. While oils are not a noteworthy source of vitamins and minerals, they do provide a significant source of energy due to their high caloric density. Extra virgin olive oil is the highest of the oils in monounsaturated fats (and the tastiest, in my opinion!). Many people use vegetable oil (which does not taste nearly as good) instead of olive oil, because they believe it is healthier. Just because the word "vegetable" is used, does not give that specific oil any magical properties. Vegetable oil is actually highest in polyunsaturated fatty acids, which are less stable in high-temperature cooking compared to monounsaturated fatty acids.[272] Only small amounts of antioxidants are found within vegetable oils, and when used during cooking with high temperatures, the molecules can become unstable and potentially release compounds that can be harmful to you, such as 4-hydroxy-*trans*-2-nonenal (HNE), which is incorporated into fried foods. [273] On the contrary, even when olive oil is heated, it remains stable and contains good levels of antioxidants. Extra virgin olive oil is considered to be the most stable of the oils when heated.[274] When olive oil is not heated, it contains more antioxidant properties than vitamin E itself!

---

272 Jessica Caporusciom, "What Are the Most Healthful Oils?," *Medical News Today*, March 30, 2019.

273 Ibid; Sarah Moumtaz et al., "Toxic Aldehyde Generation in and Food Uptake from Culinary Oils during Frying Practices: Peroxidative Resistance of a Monounsaturate-Rich Algae Oil," *Scientific Reports* 9, no. 1 (March 2019): 4125.

274 Guillaume C. De Alzaa F. and Ravetti L., "Evaluation of Chemical and Physical Changes in Different Commercial Oils During Heating," *Acta Scientific Nutritional Health* 2, no. 6 (June 2018).

The high levels of antioxidants found in olive oil can protect individuals from oxidative stress within their bodies.

POLYUNSATURATED FATS

What about the other type of "good" fat? Polyunsaturated fats are rather complex compared to monounsaturated fats. Examples of polyunsaturated fats can be found in oily fish, pine nuts, walnuts, and most of your seeds (flaxseeds, sesame seeds, sunflower seeds, and others).[275]

The two major types of polyunsaturated fats are omega-3 and omega-6 fatty acids. As if science was not confusing enough, not all omega fatty acids are polyunsaturated fatty acids. Omega-9 is actually a monounsaturated fatty acid. An example of an omega-9 fatty acid is oleic acid, which is commonly found in olive oil.[276] For the purpose of this book, we will not discuss omega-9 fatty acids in great detail.

For the Scientific Reader:

Chemically speaking, the localization of the double bond determines the type of omega fat. Omega-9 is a monounsaturated fatty acid, so it only contains one double bond, which is located nine carbons from the methyl (carbon with three hydrogen attached) end. Polyunsaturated fatty acids contain two double bonds,

---

275 Gavin Van De Walle, "Polyunsaturated Fats: Know the Facts About These Healthy Fats," *Healthline*, October 31, 2018.

276 Helda Tutunchi et al., "The Effects of Diets Enriched in Monounsaturated Oleic Acid on the Management and Prevention of Obesity: A Systematic Review of Human Intervention Studies," *Advances in Nutrition 11*, no. 4 (July 2020): 864–877.

and the placement of the first double bond is what separates them from each other. If the first double bond occurs on the third carbon atom in the chain, it is considered to be an omega-3 fatty acid, while if the first double bond occurs on the sixth carbon atom in the chain, it is considered to be an omega-6 fatty acid. Remember, this is always done by counting the carbons from the methyl end, the omega end. Omega is the last letter of the Greek alphabet. The body can synthesize omega-9 fatty acids, classifying them as non-essential fatty acids.

Omega-3 and omega-6 fatty acids are important for the structure of the membranes in your body cells and play a role in the regulation of blood pressure and inflammation.[277] It is important to understand the difference between omega-3 and omega-6 fatty acids outside of their chemical structure. Omega-6 fatty acids are commonly found in a modern diet. They can be found in vegetable oil, dairy, eggs, chicken, pork, beef, baked items (muffins, cookies, bread), and fast-food items.[278] Omega-3 fatty acids are also found in common foods, yet these foods are still not typically eaten in adequate quantities to get maximum benefits. These foods consist of fish, garlic, nuts, and seeds

277 Marc E. Surette, "The Science Behind Dietary Omega-3 Fatty Acids." *CMAJ: Canadian Medical Association Journal 178*, no. 2 (Jan 2008): 177–80.

278 "Omega-3 and Omega-6: Know the Difference," *BrainMD*, December 21, 2016.

(walnuts and chia seeds are especially high in omega-3 fatty acids).[279]

The body needs omega-6 fatty acids to survive, yet we need to minimize our dietary consumption of them. The typical American eats more omega-6 fatty acids than necessary. Many individuals are blinded by the fact that our bodies produce omega-6 fatty acids on their own. Due to the fact that they are non-essential, it is not required or recommended to eat large quantities of omega-6 fatty acids.

For the Scientific Reader:

Omega-6 fatty acids are scientifically considered to be non-essential compounds because our bodies make plenty of them. Essential compounds are unable to be synthesized from the body, making it vital to incorporate them into the diet.

Excess omega-6 fatty acids are pro-inflammatory. They cause inflammation in your body, raising your blood pressure, causing an excess of water retention, producing blood clots (which can lead to CVD), and can be linked to more severe asthma in children.[280] Omega-6 fatty acids are only bad in excess, which, unfortunately is the status of the current American diet. Omega-6 fatty acids have been shown to reduce the risks of rheumatoid arthritis, allergies, and

---

279 Ibid; "Omega-3 ALA," *California Walnuts*, accessed January 27, 2021; "Chia Seeds," *Harvard Health*, accessed January 27, 2021.

280 Emily P. Brighman et al., "Omega-3 and Omega-6 Intakes Modifies Asthma Severity and Response to Indoor Air Pollution in Children," *American Journal of Respiratory and Critical Care 199*, no. 12 (July 2019): 1478–1486.

diabetes neuropathy (a type of nerve damage in either type of diabetes caused by long-term high blood sugar).[281] There is even a correlation between omega-6 fatty acids and decreased symptoms of ADHD.[282]

Unfortunately, our bodies cannot make omega-3 fatty acids as easily as omega-6 fatty acids. This is very important to understand. Actually, the body cannot synthesize certain types of omega-3 fatty acids at all.

As complex as it already is, there are three different types of omega-3 fatty acids: Alpha-linolenic (ALA), Eicosapentaenoic acid (EPA), and Docosahexaenoic acid (DHA).[283] All three of these omega-3 fatty acids are considered to be essential and must be obtained through the diet.

For the Scientific Reader:

Through a long metabolic pathway in the body, ALA can be converted to EPA and eventually to DHA. Unfortunately, the process of converting Linoleic Acid (LA), an omega-6 polyunsaturated fatty acid, to ALA can only occur in plant desaturation. We are not plants! We must get ALA, EPA, and DHA directly from the diet, or eat enough foods high in ALA, the precursor of EPA and DHA.[284] On the flip side, LA can be converted to gamma-linoleic acid, which can be elongated and desaturated and ultimately converted to Arachidonic

---

281 "Omega-3 and Omega-6: Know the Difference," *BrainMD* (blog), December 21, 2016, accessed February 24, 2021.

282 Ibid.

283 "Omega-3 Fatty Acids," *NIH: National Institutes of Health*, last modified October 1, 2020.

284 "Ibid.

acid (AA), a polyunsaturated omega-6 fatty acid. This process is an example of the body making its own omega-6 fatty acids! AA is an important inflammatory mediator, meaning this molecule can initiate inflammatory reactions.[285] Excess omega-6 fatty acids through the diet may produce a surplus of AA, especially since the body is naturally synthesizing it as well. This may spark inflammation to arise in the body. AA is found within animal products. Simply eating one egg each day can elevate the AA levels within your blood.[286]

ALA

ALA is plant-based. Sources rich in ALA include, but are not limited to, walnuts, flaxseeds, soybeans, and others. Understanding the function of ALA may help to target neurological disorder therapy as it has anti-inflammatory properties that have shown evidence to potentially reduce the risks of strokes.[287]

Both EPA and DHA are most commonly found in cold-water fish (e.g., salmon, tuna, sardines, and others), oily fish, or other types of seafood.[288] EPA and DHA are

285 Barry Sears, *Enter the Zone: A Dietary Road Map* (New York: Regan Books, 1995).

286 Dawn, Handschuh, "Arachidonic Acid," *Nutrition Facts*, accessed January 29, 2021.

287 Nicolas Blondeau et al., "Alpha-Linolenic Acid: An Omega-3 Fatty Acid with Neuroprotective Properties—Ready for Use in the Stroke Clinic?," *Biomed Research International 2015*, (February 2015): 519830.

288 "Omega-3 Fatty Acids," *NIH: National Institutes of Health*, last modified October 1, 2020.

two essential anti-inflammatory omega-3 fatty acids that are responsible for producing resolution-phase interaction products (resolvins), which are influential inflammatory signaling molecules.[289] The name resolvins represent their role in inflammation to "resolve" it.[290]

DHA

DHA has the ability to reduce the effects of atherosclerosis by inhibiting the entry of some LDL cholesterol particles into muscle cells.[291] This is a good thing! By minimizing the amount of LDL cholesterol, the risks of developing CVD decrease.

DHA is actually the most abundant omega-3 fatty acid within the brain. This is particularly important to note as you age, because the DHA levels in your brain decline.[292] Direct associations have been reported between cognition, memory, and intelligence with DHA levels.[293] DHA may play an important role in the medical care of people who suffer from Alzheimer's disease, an irreversible progressive brain disease

---

289 Charles N Serhan et al., "Resolvins: A Family of Bioactive Products of Omega-3 Fatty Acid Transformation Circuits Initiated by Aspirin Treatment That Counter Proinflammation Signals," *The Journal of Experimental Medicine* 196, no. 8 (October 2002): 1025–37.

290 Kamal Patel, "Fish Oil," *Examine*, last modified January 6, 2021.

291 Trevor A. Mori et al., "Purified Eicosapentaenoic and Docosahexaenoic Acids Have Differential Effects on Serum Lipids and Lipoproteins, LDL Particle Size, Glucose, and Insulin in Mildly Hyperlipidemic Men," *The American Journal of Clinical Nutrition 71*, no. 5 (May 2000): 1085-1094.

292 *Puori*, "EPA and DHA Explained," June 29, 2018, video, 2:34.

293 Michael J. Weiser et al., "Docosahexaenoic Acid and Cognition throughout the Lifespan," *Nutrients 8*, no. 2 (February 2016): 99.

that strips people of their memory and cognition. Alzheimer's is very prevalent in today's society, as it affects one in ten Americans older than sixty-five.[294] Scientific research is suggesting that eating a diet with higher levels of DHA can help—DHA can heal.

Expanding off of vital brain functions, DHA plays an important role in development, especially during pregnancy and within children. In pregnancy, nutrients are transferred from the mother to the baby through the umbilical cord. DHA transferred to the baby from the mother is especially critical within the third trimester of pregnancy when the majority of brain development occurs. Without substantial levels of DHA from the mother, the baby will not have proper development of the brain, eyes, and nervous system.[295] Excellent sources of DHA during pregnancy can result in enhanced attention, behavior, and learning within children.[296] Since rapid brain growth continues during the first two years of a child's life, it is critical for newborns, infants, and toddlers (DHA is important for all ages, but especially those in the prime years of development) to adequately receive enough DHA.[297] Breast milk can be a good source of DHA; however,

---

294 "Facts and Figures," *Alzheimer's Association*, accessed January 29, 2021.

295 "3 Ways DHA Supports Moms and Babies," *OmegaQuant*, February 12, 2019.

296 Hanne Cecilie Braarud et al., "Maternal DHA Status during Pregnancy Has a Positive Impact on Infant Problem Solving: A Norwegian Prospective Observation Study," *Nutrients 10*, no. 5 (April 2018): 529; Usha Ramakrishnan et al., "Prenatal Supplementation with DHA Improves Attention at 5 Y of Age: A Randomized Controlled Trial," *The American Journal of Clinical Nutrition 104*, no. 4 (October 2016): 1075–1082.

297 *Puori*, "EPA and DHA Explained," June 29, 2018, video, 2:34.

this is dependent on the mother's intake of DHA. If you are a new mother and do not have good DHA levels or are unable to breastfeed, DHA-enriched formula does exist.[298]

Side Note:

Typically, prenatal vitamins will contain DHA and EPA to help pregnant women reach the adequate levels for themselves and their child. I will elaborate more on supplementations within the pregnant community in the supplement chapter.

EPA

EPA, your other omega-3 fatty acid, has anti-inflammatory properties, such as helping protect joints and blood vessels, which promotes faster joint recovery, a healthy heart, and overall immune function.[299] Increased EPA levels can help target inflammation that is attacking your skin. EPA can help manage oil production, reduce premature aging of the skin, and reduce acne flare ups since it is able to promote collagen production.[300] Healthy collagen is a key to healthy skin. Collagen helps to strengthen and hydrate the skin, and

---

298 University of Kansas, "DHA-Enriched Formula in Infancy Linked to Positive Cognitive Outcomes in Childhood," *ScienceDaily*, August 13, 2013.

299 *Puori*, "EPA and DHA Explained," June 29, 2018, video, 2:34.

300 Elsa H. Spencer et al., "Diet and Acne: A Review of the Evidence," *International Journal of Dermatology 48*, no. 4 (2009): 339–347; K. D. Hankenson et al., "Omega-3 Fatty Acids Enhance Ligament Fibroblast Collagen Formation in Association with Changes in Interleukin-6 Production," *Proceedings of the Society for Experimental Biology and Medicine 233*, no. 1 (January 2000): 88–95.

EPA is able to block the substance Arachidonic acid (AA) which reduces collagen output.

For the Scientific Reader:

EPA is typically thought to be better than DHA in treating inflammation. This is because EPA is able to fit into the particular enzyme of delta-5-desaturase (D5D), which produces AA.[301] Therefore, increased EPA in your diet decreases the amount of AA that is able to be produced.[302] While EPA is a better fit as an inhibitor for D5D contributing to its major anti-inflammatory role, DHA is also able to combat inflammation partially due to its own chemical inhibition ability. Refer back to the process of LA converting to Gamma-linolenic acid to eventually form AA. DHA is the inhibitor of delta-6-desaturase (D6D), an important enzyme that is the rate-limiting step of metabolizing gamma-linoleic acid. [303] Therefore, DHA can also work to limit the production of AA (gamma-linoleic acid is elongated and desaturated to form AA).

---

301 Barry Sears, *Enter the Zone: A Dietary Road Map* (New York: Regan Books, 1995).

302 Barry Sears, "What Are the Real Differences between EPA and DHA?," *Psychology Today*, April 1, 2012.

303 M. Sato et al., "Cloning of Rat Delta 6-Desaturase and Its Regulation by Dietary Eicosapentaenoic or Docosahexaenoic Acid," *World Review of Nutrition and Dietetics 88*, (2001): 196–9; D. F. Horrobin, "Fatty Acid Metabolism in Health and Disease: The Role of Delta-6-Desaturase," *The American Journal of Clinical Nutrition 57*, no. 5 (May 1993): 732S–736S.

EPA and DHA may be a potential treatment in fighting off depression.[304] This was first noticed because depression levels are lower in nations where people eat more fish, the main source of omega-3 fatty acids.[305] According to Massachusetts General Hospital and Emory University, EPA treatment may be ideal for overweight individuals who show signs of depression, and even more specifically, for those who show an abnormally high level of inflammatory activity within their body.[306] In order to control cellular inflammation in the brain, it is important to maintain high levels of EPA in the blood.[307]

For the Scientific Reader:

In order to study the depressed brain, researchers from the Tel Aviv University used the brains of genetically programmed rats to study chronic depression. The main difference highlighted high levels of AA within the brains of depressed rats. Dr. Pnina Green, the lead researcher, emphasized omega-3 fatty acids intake may reduce the levels of omega-6 AA in the

---

304 Craig Weatherby, "Omega-6 Overland Linked to Depression," *Vital Choice*, March 9, 2011.

305 David Mischoulon, "Omega-3 Fatty Acids for Mood Disorders," *Harvard Health*, last modified October 27, 2020.

306 Ibid.

307 Julian G. Martins, "EPA but Not DHA Appears to Be Responsible for the Efficacy of Omega-3 Long Chain Polyunsaturated Fatty Acid Supplementation in Depression: Evidence from a Meta-Analysis of Randomized Controlled Trials," *Journal of the American College of Nutrition 28*, no. 5 (October 2009): 525–42; Barry Sears, "What Are the Real Differences between EPA and DHA?," *Psychology Today*, April 1, 2012.

brain. As the dietary ratio of omega-6 to omega-3 fatty acids increased, so did the depressive symptoms, as the overproduction of proinflammatory cytokines, a type of signaling molecules derived from immune cells that promotes inflammation, were noted.[308] Measuring an AA/EPA or DHA ratio can be an important predictor of cellular inflammation.[309]

Omega-3 fatty acids play a vital role in reducing inflammation, which may reduce the risk of some cancers, CVD, asthma symptoms, osteoporosis (bone disease), and other conditions. According to the NIH, EPA, and DHA may even help you fend off the development of endometrial cancer![310]

So what should the ratio of EPA to DHA be? A combination is actually always preferred because this is how omega-3 fatty acids are found in nature. Doctors provide no specific ratio, because they serve different roles. You should always have levels of both in your diet, but you can learn to adjust your ratios based on your health goals (e.g., if you are looking to reduce your inflammation levels from stress, then increasing your EPA will be more beneficial). In order to protect our hearts, joints, pancreas, mood, skin, and more, we need to increase the levels of ALA, EPA, and DHA (omega-3 fatty

308 "Grants Funded," *The National Institute for Psychobiology in Israel*, accessed on March 2, 2021.

309 Valeria Tutino et al., "Elevated AA/EPA Ratio Represents an Inflammatory Biomarker in Tumor Tissue of Metastatic Colorectal Cancer Patients," *International Journal of Molecular Sciences* 20, no. 8 (April 2019): 2050.

310 "Omega-3 Fatty Acids," *National Institutes of Health*, last modified October 1, 2020.

acids) in our body from the foods that we eat because we are unable to synthesize them ourselves.[311]

SATURATED FATS

Saturated fat is referred to as the fat that is somewhere in between your "good" and "bad" fats, because it helps to increase LDL levels (this is harmful) and HDL levels (this is beneficial). Common sources of saturated fats include processed meats (burgers, ham, sausage), hard cheeses (like cheddar), whole milk and cream, butter, coconut oil, many baked goods, and other foods.[312]

For the Scientific Reader:

Within the makeup of saturated fats, "saturated" is acknowledging the hydrogen atoms that surround each carbon. Since the carbon chain in saturated fats holds hydrogen atoms at maximum capacity, it is "saturated with hydrogens."

Dating back to the 1950s, the overall popular belief was that saturated fats are bad for human health; however, current science provides no clear message.[313] Cohort studies and meta-analysis have led to contrasting conclusions despite

---

311 "The Importance of Omega-3 and Omega-6 Fatty Acids," *Eufic*, last modified March 27, 2019; Artemis P. Simopoulos, "The Importance of the Omega-6/Omega-3 Fatty Acid Ratio in Cardiovascular Disease and Other Chronic Diseases," *Experimental Biology and Medicine 233*, no. 6 (April 2008): 647–88.

312 "Saturated Fat," *Heart UK*, accessed January 29, 2021.

313 Atli Arnarson, "5 Studies on Saturated Fat- Time to Retire the Myth?," *Healthline*, February 20, 2020.

the tremendous amount of work and effort over the years dedicated to this study. In 2013, a study looked at the human health outcomes when saturated fats were replaced with LA (remember this is one of your polyunsaturated omega-6 fatty acids), such as safflower oil, a type of vegetable oil.[314] In this replacement, instead of the expected cardiovascular benefits, rates of death from CVD increased. Interestingly enough, in 2015, studying the association between saturated fat and CVD, saturated fats were replaced by carbohydrates, polyunsaturated fats, monounsaturated fats, and proteins. The only significant results occurred in the substitution with polyunsaturated fats, which appeared to be beneficial when there was a 27 percent decreased risk of CVD (excluding heart attacks, strokes, and death, in general).[315] In a similar study in 2016, replacing saturated fat with vegetable oil in an attempt to lower mortality and cholesterol levels, only resulted in an increase of cholesterol; however, it was not effective in supporting lower mortality rates.[316] Another study in 2016 researching a Dutch population found saturated fat intake is not associated with a higher risk for

314　Christopher E. Ramsden et al., "Use of Dietary Linoleic Acid for Secondary Prevention of Coronary Heart Disease and Death: Evaluation of Recovered Data from the Sydney Diet Heart Study and Updated Meta-Analysis," *BMJ 346*, (February 2013): e8707.

315　Lee Hooper et al., "Reduction in Saturated Fat Intake for Cardiovascular Disease," *The Cochrane Database of Systematic Reviews 6*, (June 2015): CD011737.

316　Christopher E. Ramsden et al., "Re-Evaluation of the Traditional Diet-Heart Hypothesis: Analysis of Recovered Data from Minnesota Coronary Experiment (1968–73)." *BMJ 353*, (April 2016): i246.

ischemic heart disease when replaced by monounsaturated and polyunsaturated fat.[317]

What is going on? I am sure you are confused, I am confused, and you know what. . . science is too. Some studies tell us that replacing saturated fats with unsaturated fats is beneficial, some claim it makes no difference, and some say that it is harmful. Science does not provide a clear understanding of the human health effects of saturated fat, which is why I classify it as an "in-between."

Although I have it classified between the two, when researching one study, I was almost convinced to move it toward the harmful side of the spectrum. From 1993 to 2011, the original Chicago Health and Aging Project (CHAP) studied over ten thousand older adults to track dementia and dietary records.[318] Within the participants, the range of saturated fats consumed was from as little as thirteen grams a day to as much as twenty-five grams a day. The study found the risk of dementia to be two to three times higher in those that consumed more saturated fats.[319] Researchers in Finland expanded off of this study by researching cognition impairments in adults (fifty years and older) to find the same pattern.[320] Most doctors, when asked

---

317   Jaike Praagman et al., "The Association between Dietary Saturated Fatty Acids and Ischemic Heart Disease Depends on the Type and Source of Fatty Acid in the European Prospective Investigation into Cancer and Nutrition–Netherlands Cohort," *The American Journal of Clinical Nutrition 103*, no. 2 (February 2016): 356–365.

318   Julia L. Bienias et al., "Design of the Chicago Health and Aging Project (CHAP)," *Journal of Alzheimer's Disease 5*, no. 5 (2003): 349–55.

319   *TedX*, "Neal Barnard: Power Foods for the Brain," September 20, 2016, video, 17:00.

320   Ibid.

about preventative actions for Alzheimer's disease will simply just explain how it is something that just happens through age and genetics. Could there really be nothing else that contributes to it? Inheriting the APOE Epsilon 4 allele can increase your risk of Alzheimer's from three (if inherited from one parent) to ten to fifteen (if inherited from both parents) times.[321] Expanding off of the Finland research study, they completed a similar study, yet candidates were only eligible if they possessed a certain genetic factor, the APOE Epsilon 4 allele. Guess what? The same results occurred. Dr. Neal Barnard, a nutrition researcher, explains that "even with the APOE Epsilon 4 allele, the risk of developing memory problems can be cut by 80 percent" if saturated fat intake is cut down.[322]

"Genes are not destiny."[323]

Being educated on the foods you consume and how they impact your health can help reduce your risk and avoid detrimental diseases such as Alzheimer's disease. While we must wait for more research to be done on saturated fat to make a decision of where to fully classify it, we do know that when eaten in moderation, saturated fat will lead to a neutral effect on blood cholesterol and when eaten in levels that are too high, saturated fat potentially can increase your risk of CVD and dementia status. [324] In the meantime, most nutritional

---

321 Ibid.

322 Ibid.

323 Ibid.

324 C. B. Dias et al., "Saturated Fat Consumption May Not Be the Main Cause of Increased Blood Lipid Levels," *Medical Hypotheses 82*, no. 2 (February 2014): 187–195.

experts recommend our saturated fat intake be limited to less than 10 percent of our daily calories.[325]

TRANS FATS

Trans fats are commonly referred to as your "bad" fats. They are the worst type of fat you can eat, because not only do they increase your LDL levels (this is harmful), but they also decrease your HDL levels (this is also harmful). Trans fats form through the process of hydrogenation, in which hydrogen is added to vegetable oil to allow solid fat to form at room temperature from a liquid.[326] Partially hydrogenated oil is the main source of artificial trans fat.[327] This is used because it is a strong preservative, meaning that it is unlikely to spoil food, which gives it a longer shelf life.

Trans fats are scientifically supported to be associated with mortality, CVD, strokes, and type II diabetes.[328] Think back to our discussion on LDL cholesterol. Fatty deposits within the arteries can block blood flow. In 2015, the Food

---

325 Katherine Zeratsky, "What's an Easy Way to See How Much Fat I Eat Each Day?," *Mayo Clinic*, May 3, 2019.

326 Charles Ophardt and Antonio Rodriguez, "Hydrogenation of Unsaturated Fats and Trans Fats," *Chemistry LibreTexts*, last modified August 10, 2020; Mayo Clinic Staff, "Trans Fat Is Double Trouble for Your Heart Health," *Mayo Clinic*, February 13, 2020.

327 "Final Determination Regarding Partially Hydrogenated Oils (Removing Trans Fats)," *FDA*, last modified May 18, 2018.

328 Russel J. de Souza et al., "Intake of Saturated and Trans Unsaturated Fatty Acids and Risk of All Cause Mortality, Cardiovascular Disease, and Type 2 Diabetes: Systematic Review and Meta-Analysis of Observational Studies," *BMJ 351*, (August 2015): h3978; Mayo Clinic Staff, "Trans Fat Is Double Trouble for Your Heart Health," *Mayo Clinic*, February 13, 2020.

and Drug Administration (FDA) determined PHOs to be no longer "Generally Recognized as Safe" (GRAS).[329] In 2018, the FDA banned all artificial trans fats in the US.[330] The US. is not the only country to ban artificial trans fats. Countries such as Denmark, Switzerland, Canada, the UK, and many more follow this trend of banning or limiting trans fats.[331] *The New York Times* predicts artificial trans fats will be eliminated worldwide by 2023.[332]

The FDA and the Institute of Medicine recommend to absolutely minimize your trans fats intake.[333] In reality, no one should eat more than two grams of trans fats a day if you are following a two thousand-calorie daily diet.[334] The FDA allows food to be declared with "no trans fats" if the food contains less than 0.5 grams of trans fat per serving (in Canada, the cut off is 0.2 grams per serving).[335]

Therefore, even if the nutrition label states zero trans fats, if you read "hydrogenated" or "partially hydrogenated" oil in the ingredient list, there is a good chance there are trans fats there. These detrimental fatty acids can be hidden in foods,

---

329 "Final Determination Regarding Partially Hydrogenated Oils (Removing Trans Fats)," *FDA*, last modified May 18, 2018.

330 Ibid.

331 "Policies to Eliminate: Industrially-Produced Trans Fat Consumption," *World Health Organization*, 2018.

332 Andrew Jacobs, "Trans Fats Should be Eliminated Worldwide by 2023, W.H.O Says," *NyTimes*, May 14, 2018.

333 Diana R. H. Winters, "The FDA's Determination on Artificial Trans Fat: A Long Time Coming," *Health Affairs* (Blog), June 20, 2015.

334 "Ask the Doctor: Does "No Trans Fat" Really Mean No Trans Fat?," *Harvard Health*, October, 2006.

335 Ibid.

such as baked goods, frozen pizzas, and fried foods.[336] This becomes particularly dangerous, because five servings of a food with "no trans fats" but "PHO" of 0.4 grams each could put you over that limit of two grams of trans fats a day without your knowing. Try to avoid trans fats whenever possible.

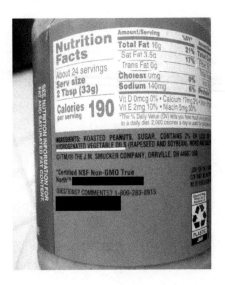

Image 1: Example of Trans Fats Hidden in Foods

For the Scientific Reader:

Triglycerides are another type of fat in the blood. High triglyceride levels are associated with an increased risk of heart attacks and strokes due to a fatty build-up in the arteries. Healthy and unhealthy fats contribute to your triglyceride levels; however, it is important

---

336   Mayo Clinic Staff, "Trans Fat Is Double Trouble for Your Heart Health," *Mayo Clinic*, February 13, 2020.

to recognize that not only can an increase in "bad" fats elevate triglyceride levels, but so can a decrease in "good" fats.[337] Your "good" fats, monounsaturated and polyunsaturated fats, help decrease LDL levels and increase HDL levels.

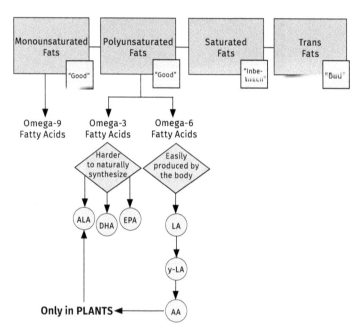

Image 2: Summary of Relationship Between the Fats.[338]

---

337 "HDL (Good), LDL (Bad) Cholesterol and Triglycerides," *American Heart Association*, last modified November 6, 2020.

338 "Omega-3 Fatty Acids," *NIH: National Institutes of Health*, last modified October 1, 2020; Nicolas Blondeau et al., "Alpha-Linolenic Acid: An Omega-3 Fatty Acid with Neuroprotective Properties—Ready for Use in the Stroke Clinic?," *Biomed Research International 2015*, (February 2015): 519830.

THE KETOGENIC DIET:

The ketogenic (keto) diet, the "most-Googled diet" of 2018, is a prime example of using fats to heal. [339] The foundation of the keto diet relies on a strict low-carbohydrate diet with an increased consumption of fats. Naturally, the body will rely on sugars (remember these are your carbohydrates) as fuel. When your body can no longer be fueled by sugars, it relies on fats. The liver will convert fatty acids to molecules called ketones, hence the name of the diet. The keto diet is one of the most controversial diets, because ketones are toxic substances and only substitute for glucose in the brain when the body is deprived of carbohydrates. This is not always recommended or considered healthy to some individuals; however, there has been great scientific research between the keto diet and epilepsy. Beta-hydroxybutyrate (BHB), a major ketone, has shown potential in being a more efficient source of fuel to the brain than glucose. The reason is that BHB provides more energy per unit of oxygen used.[340] Since seizures involve the exhaustion of energy storage in the brain (typically from an abnormal neuronal discharge), proper brain function is dependent on having enough oxygen.[341] If evidence shows that BHB can fulfill this more efficiently, then the keto diet can be declared to be an epilepsy treatment.[342]

---

339 Bailey King, "Unsurprisingly, the Ketogenic Diet Was the Most-Googled Diet in 2018," *Philly Voice*, December 18, 2018.

340 Shelly Fan, "The Fat-Fueled Brain: Unnatural or Advantageous?," *Scientific American* (blog), October 1, 2013.

341 Heng Yang et al., "Glycolysis in Energy Metabolism During Seizures," *Neural Regeneration Research 8*, no. 14 (May 2013): 1316–1326.

342 David Perlmutter, *Grain Brain: The Surprising Truth about Wheat, Carbs, and Sugar—Your Brain's Silent Killers* (New York: Little, Brown and Company, 2013).

I am not encouraging my readers to go on a keto diet. I am simply just sharing ways that food has been used to heal. It is always important to consult a doctor when deciding to make a serious diet change, and in this case, especially if you struggle with diabetes. In diabetes, not enough insulin is produced to utilize glucose to fuel the body. Due to this process, the body may force excess ketones to build up in the blood, which can be poisonous to the body, hence the term for a complication in diabetes is "ketoacidosis."[343]

Now, I want you to close your eyes and envision the first thing that comes to mind when you hear the word "fat." Has it changed? I hope it has.

---

343 "DKA (Ketoacidosis) & Ketones," *American Diabetes Association*, accessed January 27, 2021.

SIX

DAIRY

The definition of dairy according to Merriam Webster's Dictionary is "milk from a cow or other domestic animal (such as a goat); *also*: food (such as ice cream, cheese, or yogurt) made primarily of or from milk." Many people think eggs are included with dairy, but they are not.[344]

After researching dairy, I discovered two important facts. The first fact is that "milk is not necessary for humans after weaning and the nutrients it contains are available in foods without animal protein, saturated fat, and cholesterol," according to Amy Joy Lanou.[345] The second fact is that, according to the National Institutes of Health (NIH), "approximately 65 percent of the human population has a reduced ability to digest lactose after infancy."[346] This is very interesting, right?

---

344 *Merriam-Webster*, s.v. "Dairy (n.)," accessed February 19, 2021.

345 Amy Joy Lanou, "Should Dairy Be Recommended as Part of a Healthy Vegetarian Diet? Counterpoint," *The American Journal of Clinical Nutrition 89*, no. 5 (May 2009): 1638S–1642S.

346 "Lactose Intolerance," *Medline Plus*, last modified August 18, 2020.

I read that there are some studies indicating a connection to dairy and acne. I started thinking that I could have some form of dairy sensitivity. I knew something was off in my body when my acne medications continued to fail me. My acne was my sign of inflammation telling me to restore my relationship with my gut microbiome. I decided to experiment with dairy as my first step and eliminated cow milk from my diet. Within a short period of time, I noticed significant changes, suggesting milk to be a culprit of my inflammation. While this made me happy, I couldn't help but question the status of my bone health. Since osteoporosis runs in my family, would cutting my dairy intake make me more susceptible to the disease?

I was really interested in learning more about how dairy affects the body. I was surprised to discover that a lot of the things I was taught were not necessarily true. I thought milk was considered to be the golden ticket for strong bones. Actually, as long as you have a nutritious diet and include calcium from other sources, your bones will be healthy with a low-dairy diet. The debate between whether milk is the best source of calcium is still a popular discussion today. Calcium is a necessary mineral for life. Its major body source is found in our bones and teeth, which accounts for 99 percent of the calcium in our body.[347] The remaining 1 percent can be found within your body fluids, such as blood.[348] Calcium can help initiate everyday cellular function, such as muscle

---

347 "The Nutrition Source: Calcium," *Harvard Health*, accessed February 10, 2021.

348 Ibid.

contractions and is fundamental for the structural integrity of your skeleton backbone.[349]

It is crucial to obtain adequate levels of calcium from within your diet. Without enough calcium, your body will be forced to take calcium from its major supplier: your bones. An overabundant "borrowing" of calcium from the bones can lead to osteoporosis, a condition where bone mass will decrease, and bones become weak and brittle.[350] Other chronic conditions due to calcium deficiency (hypocalcemia) include mood disorders (anxiety, depression, and others), heart problems, tooth decay, and inadequate blood clotting.[351]

For the Scientific Reader:

Le Châtelier's Principle can chemically explain how the body is able to "borrow" calcium concentrations from within the bones.

Calcium is not only needed for healthy bones and teeth, but also for chemical messages, blood clotting, muscle contraction, and heart rhythm regulation.[352] Refer to the chart below to see the Institute of Medicine's (IOM) daily recommended calcium intake levels.[353] Note that the highest

---

349 "General Chemistry Lab Tutorials: Calcium in the Body," *Washington University St. Louis*, accessed February 3, 2021.

350 "Calcium and Bone Health," *Help Guide*, last modified October 2020.

351 Ibid.

352 "General Chemistry Lab Tutorials: Calcium in the Body," *Washington University St. Louis*, accessed February 3, 2021.

353 "Calcium and Your Child," *John Hopkins Medicine*, accessed February 3, 2021.

recommended intake occurs between the ages of nine to eighteen. This is due to puberty hormones being produced during adolescence, which are responsible for speeding up bone growth.[354] Keep in mind that women may need to consume more than the daily calcium recommendations. Women have a higher risk of osteoporosis since the calcium balance in the body can be affected by different hormones, physical activity, vitamin D, and diet, which all may differ by individual, but can also be impacted by sex.[355]

Age:	IOM Recommended Daily Calcium Intake (milligrams)
Adult	1,000
9 - 18 years old	1,300
4 - 8 years old	1,000
1 - 3 years old	700

Table 1: The Institute of Medicine's daily calcium intake recommendations.

It is commonly believed that milk is the best source of calcium. Growing up I never had a problem with drinking milk but my brother, Sam, refused to drink it, which challenged my parents. How were they going to get Sam to grow big and tall like my dad who is 6'2"? It was not until Sam discovered strawberry milk that my parents felt at ease with their children's calcium intake. Sam drank strawberry milk

---

354 Luiz Claudio Castro et al., "Children and Bone Health," *Hormone Health Network*, last modified July 2020

355 "General Chemistry Lab Tutorials: Calcium in the Body," *Washington University St. Louis*, accessed February 3, 2021.

almost every day and was able to surpass my dad's height by his freshman year in college. The question now comes down to would Sam have been able to grow to be 6'3" if he never got hooked on strawberry milk? If Sam never incorporated milk into his diet what would his bone health be like?

The average glass of milk contains around three hundred milligrams of calcium.[356] If, for some reason the nutrition label only provides you with the daily percentage value, you can simply add a zero to the end of this number to find out an estimate of how many milligrams of calcium it contains.[357] For example, 30 percent of your daily calcium requirement would be around three hundred milligrams. However, bear in mind that you are always absorbing slightly less than the value given on the nutrition label. Donna Herock, MD, and spokeswoman for the Physicians Committee for Responsible Medicine, states "When you eat a protein food, such as milk, you may be swallowing calcium, but you turn around and excrete calcium in your urine."[358]

Although milk proteins may eliminate some of the calcium from milk, milk still remains a great source of calcium. Connie Weaver, PhD, the head of foods and nutrition at Purdue University, emphasizes that drinking milk causes more calcium to enter the body than to be excreted.[359] Each glass of milk provides around eight grams of protein and thee hundred milligrams of calcium. Within each gram of

356 "Calcium Content of Foods," *UCSF Health*, accessed February 11, 2021.

357 "Increasing Calcium in Your Diet," *Cleveland Clinic*, last modified December 1, 2019.

358 "Milk for Your Bones?," *WebMD*, October 6, 2000.

359 Ibid.

protein 1.75 milligrams of calcium is lost. [360] Therefore, in each glass of milk you will lose approximately fourteen out of three hundred milligrams of calcium. While milk remains a good source of calcium, is it the best?

Three hundred milligrams of calcium are easier to obtain than you may have been taught. A glass of fortified orange juice and a cup of dried figs both contain three hundred milligrams of calcium.[361] There are many other foods that are considered to be great sources of calcium: whole almonds (385 milligrams per cup), baked beans (127 milligrams per serving), broccoli (72 milligrams per serving), one cup of bok choy (159 milligrams), chia seeds (179 milligrams per two tablespoons), collard greens (226 milligrams per serving), one cup of edamame (68 milligrams per cup), kale (94 milligrams per serving), a large orange (74 milligrams), sardines, canned with bones (325 milligrams), a cup of spinach (250 milligrams), and so many more.[362] Even soy and nut milks are often fortified to the same or greater levels of calcium than cow milk. All of the food items I just mentioned are dairy-free, so if you struggle with lactose intolerance, do not feel deterred from obtaining adequate calcium levels.

For the Scientific Reader:

Similar to how proteins may affect calcium absorption in dairy products, phytates found in plant-derived foods, and oxalates found in green leafy vegetables can affect the bioavailability of calcium. Phytates may block some of the calcium absorption and oxalates

360 Ibid.

361 Ibid.

362 Ibid.

can bind to calcium, also preventing some absorption. However, plant-based foods, such as the ones listed above, still prove to be an adequate calcium source. The main takeaway is there are many non-dairy foods that provide sufficient calcium levels.

The debate between whether milk is the best source of calcium is still a popular discussion today. Dairy supporters will claim milk is perfect in transporting calcium to bones in adequate levels, while non-dairy supporters claim milk robs calcium from bones and will support plant-based foods to provide a better choice. Turns out Sam would have been able to reach the height of 6'3" and have healthy bones without his strawberry milk, but only if he was getting an adequate source of calcium from other foods.

LACTOSE INTOLERANCE

The Physicians Committee for Responsible Medicine stresses for "there to be no reason for people with lactose intolerance to push themselves to drink milk."[363] Over five billion people in the world have a reduced ability to digest lactose after infancy (this is 65 percent of the world's population).[364]

Most dairy foods contain lactose, a natural sugar. In fact, only a few dairy items are composed of little to no lactose, such as hard cheese.[365] Dr. Daniel Cramer, OBGYN, with the Brigham and Women's Hospital in Boston, believes lactose

363 "Can People Who Are Lactose Intolerant Consume Milk Anyway?," *Pro-Con*, last modified April 9, 2008.

364 "Lactose Intolerance," *Medline Plus*, last modified August 18, 2020.

365 "What is the Lactose Content of Different Dairy Products?," *Dairy Australia*, last modified September 18, 2019.

sugar may be responsible for infertility. Women are most fertile in their twenties; however, many are not ready to start a family until much later due to career focuses.[366] When they are older, many women are reminded by their doctors and family members that their childbearing time is of the essence, since fertility rates significantly decrease with age. There is a notable difference between fertility rates of a woman in her late twenties versus late thirties. Dr. Cramer investigated this concept by comparing those fertility rates in women across numerous countries that consist of various diets. The ten-year difference resulted in a 25 percent fertility decrease in Thailand, where dairy does not constitute a major part of their diet. Brazil, a country with a mild dairy consumption, yielded a 50 percent decrease in fertility. A high dairy consumption country, like the US, reported an 80 percent decrease in fertility.[367] Dr. Cramer believes the culprit of this dilemma is due to the lactose sugar itself. Lactose is a disaccharide, meaning it consists of two sugar subunits, composed of glucose and galactose. The "mammalian ovary is particularly susceptible to damage from the accumulation of galactose and galactose metabolites."[368] Galactose can be toxic to the ovaries.

Dairy is the most common food intolerance. There are many different types of lactose intolerances and sensitivities

---

366 *Physicians Committee*, Neal Barnard, MD: How Food Affects Hormones, March 18, 2020, video, 54:19.

367 Daniel W. Cramer et al., "Adult Hypolactasia, Milk Consumption, and Age-Specific Fertility," *American Journal of Epidemiology 139*, no. 3 (1994): 282–9.

368 G Liu et al., "Galactose Metabolism and Ovarian Toxicity," *Reproductive Toxicology 14*, no. 5 (September-October 2000): 377-84.

that may be developed. The most common type, being primary lactose intolerance, which is when the amount of lactase enzyme being made is decreased through time (this is lactase non-persistence and it is a normal result of aging).[369]

Secondary lactose intolerance may result from an injury to the small intestine or from an illness such as celiac disease (refer to the gluten chapter) or inflammatory bowel disease (Crohn's disease and ulcerative colitis, causing chronic inflammation in the gastrointestinal tract). However, this type of intolerance may not be permanent. If the underlying illness is treated, then lactase enzyme levels may normalize.[370] In some rare cases, you can be born with a lactose intolerance (congenital lactose intolerance), which may be life-threatening, since the baby will not be able to digest breast milk.[371] In this type of intolerance, there is a complete absence of the lactase enzyme from an inherited autosomal recessive pattern (meaning you must inherit a mutated gene from each parent).[372] Many other types of lactose intolerance/sensitivity exist.

I was able to chat with Dr. Darwin Deen, a nutritionist, educator, and author of *Nutrition for Life*. One of the first questions I asked Dr. Deen was why he became interested in nutrition.

His answer resonated with me. Dr. Deen was around fourteen years old when he started experiencing daily discomfort in two areas of his body: his head and his stomach. Similar to my acne, he struggled to find the appropriate

---

369 Mayo Clinic Staff, "Lactose Intolerance," *Mayo Clinic*, April 7, 2020.

370 Ibid.

371 "Lactose Intolerance," *Medline Plus*, last modified August 18, 2020.

372 Ibid.

treatment. Not only did he feel discomfort in his abdominal region, but he experienced borborygmi, which essentially is what you would think of when you are hungry and your stomach "growls." His body was blatantly trying to communicate with him to restore his relationship with his gut microbiome. Borborygmi is a normal part of digestion, aiding in the travel of food, liquid, and gas between the stomach and small intestines, but excess levels are directly related to either hunger or indigestion. Unfortunately, he and his doctors looked past these obvious signs and tried to treat his conditions with eyeglasses (in the belief that his headaches were caused by vision impairments) and therapy (in the belief that his indigestion was caused by aerophagia (swallowing too much air) associated with neurosis (a stress-related mental illness)). Continually being misdiagnosed, Dr. Deen learned to live with his discomfort for years, as millions of people do.

It is scary to feel off-sync with your body, to know that something is wrong, and have professional after professional misdiagnose your symptoms. When Dr. Deen was in his final year of college, he decided to enroll in a nutrition class. Little did Dr. Deen know how much this course and the professor would change his life. His "aha" moment occurred during a class devoted to lactose intolerance, one of the most common nutritional problems in the world. It was not until every single symptom of lactose intolerance was listed out that Dr. Deen realized his condition. "I fell off my chair," he stated.

Imagine the joy that rushed across Dr. Deen when he realized that he was not crazy and that he could actually cure his discomfort. This is how I felt when I realized I could use food to help treat my chronic acne.

"No doctor had ever asked
me about my diet."

- DR. DARWIN DEEN

Dr. Deen was lactose intolerant his entire life, but he was unaware of it. Once this discovery was made, Dr. Deen was able to experiment with his intolerance and listen to his body as to what exact dairy products made him feel sicker than others. His key discovery actually revolved around the idea of fat. Dr. Deen realized that he had no issues digesting most dairy products (excluding milk) if it had enough fat in it.

According to the NIH US National Library of Medicine, "Most people with lactase nonpersistence retain some lactase activity and can include varying amounts of lactose in their diets without experiencing symptoms. Often, affected individuals have difficulty digesting fresh milk but can eat certain dairy products such as cheese or yogurt without discomfort. These foods are made using fermentation processes that break down much of the lactose in milk."[373]

To reiterate, lactose intolerance results from decreased lactase enzymes in the body that make it difficult to break down lactose from dairy products. Since fat slows down peristalsis (the movement through your gut), dairy products high in fat can allow the minimal amount of lactase enzymes in the body to have more time to break down the lactose in dairy. This may only be true in the cases of those individuals with specific types of lactose intolerances where they still have amounts of lactase enzymes. In Dr. Deen's case, he has

---

373 Ibid.

minimal to no issues with half and half cream, ice cream, and full fat yogurt; however, a simple glass of skim milk will cause him to experience extreme symptoms of lactose intolerance. If you are lactose intolerant/sensitive, it is important to keep in mind that just because you can tolerate fatty dairy products does not mean they are beneficial for you. Fatty dairy products have been associated with increased risk of cardiovascular disease (CVD) and mortality.[374] Fatty dairy products are considered a high energy-dense food, meaning there are a lot of calories in a small quantity due to their high content of carbohydrates, sugars, and fats. A healthier and delicious substitute for ice cream is full-fat yogurt!

Side note: Erectile Dysfunction

In discussing erectile dysfunction, Dr. Neal Barnard, former psychiatrist and founder of the Barnard Medical Center emphasizing preventative medicine and diet, discusses that a good doctor will prescribe the patient Viagra, but a great doctor will explain that his issues may not be solely derived from performance anxiety, but maybe from atherosclerosis. Atherosclerosis refers to the narrowing of the arteries from excess fat and cholesterol. Since the most narrowed arteries originally are the ones that stem down to the private parts, it is common to first experience poor

---

374 Carole Davis and Etta Saltos, Dietary Recommendations and How They Have Changed Over Time," *Economic Research Service, U.S. Department of Agriculture,* 33–50; Javier Fontecha et al., "Milk and Dairy Product Consumption and Cardiovascular Diseases: An Overview of Systematic Reviews and Meta-Analyses," *Advances in Nutrition 10,* no. 2 (May 2019): S164–S189.

blood flow in those areas. It only takes a matter of time for the arteries to restrict the heart and brain, putting erectile dysfunction patients at a higher risk for heart attacks and strokes. A great doctor may prescribe Viagra, but they will also explain how to use food to reverse the atherosclerosis that could kill you.[375] It is important to not just watch out for the milks that are high in fat, but also for most cheeses, which are 70 percent fat (mostly saturated fat, which we know can be harmful).[376]

Now, I'm going to share information about kefir and yogurt, two different types of fermented milk consisting of different yeast and bacteria cultures, which have been found to improve lactose digestion by 54 to 71 percent compared to the average milk.[377,378]

FERMENTED FOODS

Foods like cheese and yogurt are made using fermentation processes, which break down most of the lactose found in

---

375 *Physicians Committee*, Neal Barnard, MD: How Food Affects Hormones, March 18, 2020, video, 54:19.

376 "Health Concerns About Dairy," *Physicians Committee for Responsible Medicine*, accessed February 11, 2021.

377 Abbott Laboratories, "Kefir Improves Lactose Digestion and Tolerance in Adults with Lactose Digestion," *Journal of the American Dietetic Association 103*, no. 5 (May 2003): 582–7.

378 Damiana D Rosa et al., "Milk Kefir: Nutritional, Microbiological and Health Benefits," *Nutrition Research Reviews 30*, no. 1 (February 2017): 82–96.

milk.[379] The lower levels in lactose help explain one of the reasons why fermented dairy products are easier for a lactose intolerant/sensitive person to digest. Fermented foods may help those who suffer from lactose-intolerance, irritable bowel syndrome (IBS), Crohn's disease, and type II diabetes to have an easier time digesting dairy food.[380]

KEFIR

Kefir, which resembles a smoothie (due to its thick texture), is made by mixing milk proteins and grain-like live yeast and bacteria cultures and allowing it to ferment for twenty-four hours.[381] The key ingredient of kefir is the kefir grains.[382] If you want to try kefir, you can find it at the local grocery store in the dairy aisle.

There are many types of kefir and experimenting with different brands will help you find one that suits your taste. Remember, if you are lactose intolerant and are thinking of trying this, it is always a good idea to consult your doctor. . . and listen to your body. Make sure to always pay attention to how your body reacts to what you put in it. Everyone has different reactions to different foods, and these are just some tips and tricks that may be able to help you.

YOGURT

The more commonly known and consumed fermented dairy is yogurt. A multitude of scientific evidence reveals yogurt

---

379   "Lactose Intolerance," *Medline Plus*, last modified August 18, 2020.

380   Ronan Lordan et al., "Dairy Fats and Cardiovascular Disease: Do We Really Need to Be Concerned?," *Foods* 7, no. 3 (May 2018): 29.

381   Ibid.

382   Ibid.

to benefit human health. Yogurt can help aid in gastrointestinal issues, such as diarrhea.[383] There are so many different types, flavors, and brands of yogurt. Are they all proven to be associated with positive human health outcomes? How do you find the best yogurt for you?

It is well-known that many yogurts contain probiotics. Have you ever noticed your doctor recommending that you increase the amount of probiotics in your diet, from foods like yogurt, when you are on antibiotic medications? This is because, unfortunately when antibiotics kill off bad bacteria in your body, they also cause collateral damage to some good bacteria in your body. Increasing your probiotic intake can replenish some of the good bacteria. Different types of yogurt may contain different types of probiotic strains, some better than others, but two strains will always remain the same. The strains of *Lactobacillus bulgaricus* (L. bulgaricus) and *Streptococcus thermophilus* (S. thermophilus*) are required by the US Code of Federal Regulations to be present in all yogurts due to their significant ability to help digest lactose.[384]

There are many other examples of different probiotic strains, but just to highlight one, the popular yogurt company Dannon specifically designed the yogurt brand Activia to incorporate an additional strain of probiotics,

383 P. Glibowski and A. Turczyan, "Determining the Effect of Consuming Fermented Milk Drinks on the Incidence of Constipation, Diarrhoea and Resistance to Respiratory Illness," *Roczniki Państwowego Zakładu Higieny 64*, no. 4 (2013).

384 "Yogurt," *Harvard Health*, accessed February 4, 2021; "Yogurt Production," *Milk Facts*, accessed February 4, 2021.

Bifidobacterium lactis.[385] The French scientist Denis Guy-onne studied this probiotic strain and reported improvement in indigestion and IBS symptoms in yogurts with added *Bifidobacterium lactis.*[386]

When buying yogurt it is important to ensure it contains at least one hundred million cultures per gram at manufacture time or at least ten million cultures per gram for frozen yogurts, which is what is required to consider yogurt healthy according to the International Dairy Foods Association (IDFA) [387] This information can be found on the *Live and Active Cultures* (LAC) seal on yogurts.

While yogurt is linked to increasing the good bacteria in your gut, not all yogurts are as healthy as you were led to believe. Similar to fruit containing the natural sugar of fructose, yogurt (and other dairy products as well) contains natural sugars of lactose. However, many yogurt brands include additives, such as added sugar, gelatin, and artificial colors/flavors to increase the palatability and flavors of their products. Please refer back to the added sugar section within the inflammation chapter if you need a refresher on the negative health effects associated with these. When reading the food labels on yogurts, it is advised to choose a yogurt that has less than fifteen grams of sugar per serving.[388]

---

385 Jacquelyn Cafasso, "10 Reasons to Take a Bifidus Probiotic," *Healthline*, last modified October 12, 2017.

386 Ibid.

387 "Live & Active Cultures Seal," *International Dairy Foods Association (IDFA)*, accessed February 4, 2021.

388 Megan Ware, "Everything You Need to Know about Yogurt," *Medical News Today*, January 11, 2018.

It may be more challenging to determine the added sugar content in yogurts than originally thought, since many food labels only list total sugars, without a breakdown. This provides no clarity in knowing how many grams of those sugars are from added sugars. Katherine Isacks, a dietitian and certified diabetes educator, shows how you could calculate the amounts of added sugars, if you desire.[389] To do this, subtract the number of grams of sugar in the fruit flavor versus the plain yogurt of the same brand. Be sure to check if the yogurts have the same serving size. Unfortunately, plain yogurts and flavored yogurts often are sold with different serving sizes. An unflavored plain Greek yogurt typically has zero grams of added sugars. Keep in mind that flavors such as blueberry, strawberry, and vanilla are typically sweetened with added sugars. If you prefer flavored yogurt, try adding your own honey, fruit, or other flavorings to plain yogurt. This way you are able to control how much added sugar goes into what you are eating.

Besides kefir and yogurt, additional fermented dairy products include: filmjölk, cultured cream, certain fresh cheeses, sour cream, and natural buttermilk.

PROTEIN CONTENT

Nicole Dynan, a dietitian and expert in gut health, highlights the benefit of dairy milk due to its high protein content.[390] In comparing the protein levels of a full-fat/whole milk Greek yogurt to a similar branded coconut yogurt, the full fat yogurt has around sixteen grams of protein, while

389 "Katherine Isacks," *My Net Diary,* accessed February 4, 2021.

390 "Gut Feelings: The Power of Fermented Dairy," *The Guardian, Dairy Australia,* accessed February 4, 2021.

the coconut yogurt has one or less grams of protein.[391] This is a major difference that people often do not take into consideration very often. Dr. Deen emphasizes the importance of having protein in his meals, and since he eats yogurt for breakfast, he emphasizes how it does not make sense for him to make the substitution from full-fat yogurt to one that is low-fat.

This is important to keep in mind when following the latest trend of nut milks. The protein levels vary greatly between nut and cow milks. Cow milk provides around eight grams of protein per cup, while most nut milks only contain one gram of protein per cup: almond (one gram) coconut (zero grams), and oat (two grams). [392]

Side note:

Soy milk is an exception in the protein trend of non-cow milk, since it contains seven to eight grams of protein!

In regard to almond milk, it is important to keep an eye out for the word "Carrageenan" on its nutrition label. Many almond milks contain Carrageenans, which are derived from seaweed and help thicken and stabilize foods; however, it has not been adequately tested and some studies have shown that

391 "Coconut-Based Vanilla," *Chobani*, accessed February 13, 2021; "Whole Milk Plain Greek Yogurt," *Chobani*, accessed February 13, 2021.

392 Liza Torborg, "Mayo Clinic Q and A: Dairy Milk, Soy Milk, Almond Milk – Which is the Healthiest Choice for you?," *Mayo Clinic: News Network*, April 9, 2019; "Unsweetened Almond Milk," *Califia Farms*, accessed February 13, 2021; "Coconut Milk," *Califia Farms*, accessed February 13, 2021; "Oat Milk," *Califia Farms*, accessed February 13, 2021.

it contributes to gastrointestinal discomfort and inflammation symptoms.[393]

Nut milk is very different from cow milk. Nut milk is made by blending nuts and water. The composition of nut milks greatly differs from cow milks. Although both are a great source of calcium (nut milks are fortified to the same level as cow milks) I am not sure who decided to name and classify these beverages as milks because based on its ingredients it should be called nut waters. When drinking nut milk, it is important to ask yourself, "Why?" If it is for lactose sensitivity and inflammation issues, nut milks will be your friend; however, if you want a good source of protein, you should stick to cow milk.

HORMONES:

There is no such thing as hormone-free milk. Even cows that are not injected with bovine growth hormones (which are FDA-approved drugs that are used to increase milk production)[394] still produce hormone milk. Cows are impregnated annually. The gestation period for a cow range averages 283 days, meaning for around nine to twelve months a year, cows are pregnant and producing estrogen.[395] Estrogen is able to travel from the blood plasma into the milk. Similar to all hormones, you are looking for that sweet spot, since too much and too little quantities may be fatal. However, unlike other hormones, estrogen can enter the cell membrane, sneak into

---

393 Kathleen Pointer, "Should You Remove Carrageenan from Your Diet?," *Healthline*, last modified October 12, 2017.

394 "Bovine Somatotropin (bST)," *FDA*, last modified April 21, 2020.

395 "Pregnant Cows, Timing of Pregnancy, Open Cows, Pregnancy Rate," *Institute of Agriculture and Natural Resources*, accessed February 10, 2021.

the nuclear membrane (also known as the nuclear envelope) and can result in rapid cell production as it can attach and manipulate DNA.

Studies have been able to link higher blood estrogen levels with postmenopausal breast cancer. Around 80 percent of all breast cancers are reported to emerge from estrogen supplies.[396]

For the Scientific Reader:

It confuses many people that high estrogen intensifies the risks of breast cancer, but peaks in breast cancer prevalence occur ten to twenty years post-menopause. Aren't these concepts contradictory? Turns out when ovaries halt the production of estrogen, it's dependent on local sources directly in the breasts. Additionally, estrogen can be made in local levels in fat, and overall excess fat in the body can signal the gene aromatase, which is responsible for the biosynthesis of estrogens.[397] Unfortunately, science is not sure why estrogen increases the risks of breast cancer. Some theorized this relates back to the fact that estrogen can sneak into the nuclear membrane and potentially help produce cancerous cells by speeding up the multiplication process.[398] Estrogen is a natural

396 Sarah Brechon, "Estrogen and Breast Cancer," *Maurer Foundation: Breast Health Education*, February 7, 2012.

397 *Breast Cancer Research Foundation*, "If Most Breast Cancers Are Driven by Estrogen, Why Are Peak Incidences after Menopause?," April 10, 2014, video, 1:10.

398 Sarah Brechon, "Estrogen and Breast Cancer," *Maurer Foundation: Breast Health Education*, February 7, 2012.

steroid hormone found in both men and women. So, to bust the myth that men can't get breast cancer: yes, it is possible.

MALE FERTILITY:

Do not be fooled to the common reference of estrogen as "women hormones." Men still have plentiful estrogen levels. In a study to look at estrogen's effects on male fertility, the sperm count was compared between men who ate a lot of cheese compared to those who barely ate it. Remember, cheese is derived from milk, which comes from cows, so it contains hormones, as well. The results showed that even traces of estrogen in milk and cheese are potentially able to strip a man of his fertility. The sperm count of the men whose diet consisted of a lot of cheese was significantly less than those who ate little cheese.[399] Surprisingly, this study claimed that estrogen may not be the sole factor as to why this is the case. Other theories believe these effects may be due to environmental contaminants within the milk/cheese, such as pesticides.[400] This makes us wonder if certain dairy products may be even worse than what we think?

SOY

In 1931, the isoflavone, Genestine, was discovered in soy. Genestine is presented in a very similar manner to estrogen

399 *Physicians Committee*, Neal Barnard, MD: How Food Affects Hormones, March 18, 2020, video, 54:19.

400 M. Afeiche et al., "Dairy Food Intake in Relation to Semen Quality and Reproductive Hormone Levels among Physically Active Young Men," *Human Reproduction 28*, no. 8 (August 2013): 2265–2275.

and actually binds to the same receptor. Since most breast cancers arise with high estrogen levels, when Genestine is able to compete and bind to the same receptor it slows down cancer growth. Soy food consumption has shown a significant relationship in decreasing the risk of death and cancer recurrence.[401] Switching out dairy milk for soy milk can have many positive effects, especially regarding your relationship with breast cancer. Keep in mind that milk is not hormone free and contains levels of estrogen. Even if it is a trace amount, it makes a difference. Other good sources of soy include tofu, edamame, and miso.[402]

ACNE AND DAIRY

Estrogen is not the only hormone found in milk. The most prominent androgens, testosterone and androstenedione, are included in milk as well.[403] While you may know these as "male hormones," do not be deceived. They are actually present in higher quantities than estrogens in women.[404] One of the many reasons as to why milk may cause acne is due to its androgenic components. Testosterone prompts sebum production. Sebum is an oily substance created by sebaceous glands beneath the skin, which is present in the largest concentration on your face. When these glands become blocked,

---

401 Xiao Ou Shu et al., "Soy Food Intake and Breast Cancer Survival," *JAMA* *302*, no. 22 (December 2010): 2437–2443.

402 "A Guide to Foods Rich in Soy," *UCSF Health*, accessed February 10, 2021.

403 Clement A. Adebamowo et al., "High School Dietary Dairy Intake and Teenage Acne," *Journal of the American Academy of Dermatology 52*, no. 2 (February 2005): 207–214.

404 James Simon, "Androgen," *Healthy Women*, accessed February 11, 2021.

the result is inflammation in the form of acne.[405] A surplus of testosterone over accumulates sebum, which escalates acne flare-ups. People who suffer from acne yield greater amounts of testosterone than those without acne.[406]

Side note:

If you were ever curious as to why certain birth controls may help alleviate acne inflammation, it is because the synthetic estrogen and progesterone can lower the level of androgens in your body, having an anti-androgenic effect. However, it is also important to note why some birth controls may cause acne. This is because hormones in specific birth controls may act as androgens in the body itself.

Various studies report associations of several milk types and acne. Girls aged nine to fifteen were reported more likely to have acne with cow milk (whole, low-fat, or skim) in their diet.[407] In 2008, Harvard reported boys aged nine to fifteen more likely to have acne with skim milk compared to the other milks in their diet.[408] In 2004, a correlation was found

---

405 *Dr. Davin Lim,* "Skin Care Tips- Treating Hormonal Acne," May 20, 2018, video, 13:53.

406 Evgenia Makrantonaki et al., "An Update on the Role of the Sebaceous Gland in the Pathogenesis of Acne," *Dermatoendocrinology 3*, no.1 (2011): 41–9.

407 Clement A. Adebamowo et al., "Milk Consumption and Acne in Adolescent Girls," *Dermatology Online Journal 12*, no. 4 (May 2006): 1.

408 Clement A. Adebamowo et al., "Milk Consumption and Acne in Teenaged Boys," *Journal of the American Academy of Dermatology 58*, no. 5 (2008): 787–793.

between acne in adult women and total intake of milk and skim milk from the Nurses Health Study II.[409] While there are different findings, depending on the type of milk (whole, skim, 2 percent, low-fat, etc.), most studies conducted on the topic of dairy and acne have concluded that dairy milk may be a factor in contributing to acne.

Specifically, a stronger connection has been found with skim milk when compared to other milks.[410] In addition to the presence of androgens in milk, milk proteins consist of whey and casein, which make up 20 and 80 percent, respectively, and have been linked to acne. [411] It should come as no surprise to learn that skim milk contains slightly higher levels of whey protein![412] If you struggle with acne, Dr. Wil-

409   Clement A. Adebamowo et al., "High School Dietary Dairy Intake and Teenage Acne," *Journal of the American Academy of Dermatology* 52, no. 2 (February 2005): 207–214.

410   Ibid; Clement A. Adebamowo et al., "Milk Consumption and Acne in Teenaged Boys," *Journal of the American Academy of Dermatology* 58, no. 5 (2008): 787–793.

411   Anna Haug et al., "Bovine Milk in Human Nutrition – A Review," *Lipids in Health and Disease* 6, no. 25 (September 2007); William F. Danby, "Nutrition and Acne," *Clinics in Dermatology* 28, no. 6 (November-December 2010): 598–604; Fatma Perlin Cengiz et al., "Acne Located on the Trunk, Whey Protein Supplementation: Is There Any Association?," *Health Promotion Perspectives* 7, no. 2 (March 2017): 106–108.

412   Becky Bell, "Is Whole Milk Better Than Low-Fat and Skim Milk?," *Healthline*, October 26, 2016; George Q. Chen et al., "Chapter 8 – Membrane Separations in the Dairy Industry," *Separation of Functional Molecules in Food by Membrane Technology* (2019): 267–304; Angela Palmer, The Link Between Milk and Acne," *Verywell Health*, last modified December 10, 2019.

liam Danby from the department of medicine of Dartmouth Medical School recommends staying away from milk proteins, especially in protein powders. He claims there are no reports of worse acne in people consuming soy-based protein shakes.[413]

The information embedded in our brain about milk is not as truthful as we were led to believe. Most dairy products are linked to different diseases and inflammation within our body, and over half of the world's population is sensitive to the lactose carbohydrate itself. So why is it so prevalent in our diet? Remember the further from the cow, the less adverse the effects! Fermented dairy products, such as yogurt have shown beneficial overall effects on human health and restoring our relationship with our gut microbiome. If you thought milk was the best source of calcium and contained vital nutrients that cannot be obtained elsewhere, think again. All the nutrients found in milk can be found in different products.

413   William F. Danby, "Nutrition and Acne," *Clinics in Dermatology 28*, no. 6 (November-December 2010): 598–604.

SEVEN

SUPPLEMENTS

Years ago, I had a doctor's appointment with my primary care physician. One of the first questions my doctor asked me was what medications I was taking. Without hesitating, I responded that I was only taking an oral contraceptive. Looking at my medical chart, my doctor questioned if I was still taking the topical creams prescribed by my dermatologist. Having not initially considered medications that were not in pill form, I wondered why my primary care physician cared to know if I had put a pea-sized dot of lotion on my face. Could this really make a significant impact on my health? Toward the end of our visit, my doctor double-checked that I was taking a birth control pill and using one topical cream for my acne. While my doctor had done her part, I had not done mine. That day, I failed as a patient, and even worse, I did not realize until years later that I should have shared a supplement I was taking.

My insecurities about my skin had led me to fall into false advertising and "too good to be true" marketing tactics of the supplement industry. While I don't recall if I found out about this miracle acne solution from a Google search, an Instagram post, or by word-of-mouth, I eagerly purchased a bottle and started the daily prebiotic/probiotic regime. After a month, I didn't notice a difference and did not want to spend more money on another bottle, so I stopped. However, I should have shared this information with my doctor because, contrary to popular belief, supplements are medications as well. This is vitally important because medications can interact with each other and potentially cause adverse reactions or exacerbate existing health issues. However, if doctors are aware of the entirety of medications and supplements you are taking, they can adjust treatment paradigms to avoid contraindications. My intentions were not to be secretive with my doctor. I was simply uneducated to consider supplements as a medication, and apparently, I am not the only one.

In early 2020, I heard a story of a twenty-three-year-old woman who suffered from acute liver failure, which her doctor thought could be attributed to a supplement she was taking. In hopes of fixing her chronic acne, she had taken four supplement pills a day for over ten months. During this time, she experienced fatigue, abdominal pain, and yellow discoloration of her eyes, which indicates liver dysfunction. Her doctors strongly ruled out other causes, such as jaundice, hepatitis, and auto-immune disorders, believing that she had entered a state of drug-induced acute liver failure due to the supplement.[414] While I am only mentioning one case, unfortunately, there are many more. In 2017, herbal and dietary supplements were to blame for 20 percent of

---

414 *The Doctors*, "Woman Almost Dies After Taking Daily Supplements?," February 19, 2020, video, 4:50.

the hepatotoxicity (toxicity in the liver) cases in the US.[415] Dr. Jeffrey Weinstein, gastroenterologist and the medical director of liver transplantations at the Methodist Dallas Medical Center, declared that even supplements claimed as natural and for health benefits should be viewed as chemicals and drugs.[416]

In fact, the use of dietary supplements was reported at an all-time high in 2019. The Consumer Survey on Dietary Supplements announced the consumption of dietary supplements in 77 percent of Americans. The largest users are classified as middle-aged adults (thirty-five to fifty-four years old) representing a prevalence of 81 percent.[417]

If you are taking an herbal or dietary supplement, I am not trying to convince you to stop. Not all supplements are bad and some actually have beneficial outcomes. The main takeaway is to inform your doctor so that they can take into consideration any concerns they may have.

THE TRUTH ABOUT SUPPLEMENTS

Aggressive print and internet marketing may lead people to believe that spending a certain amount of money on supplements each month will yield a healthier life. The truth is that many supplements are water-soluble, meaning

---

415   Victor Navarro et al., "Liver Injury from Herbal and Dietary Supplements," *Hepatology 65*, no. 1 (July 2017): 363–373.

416   Melkorka Licea, "Woman Says She Suffered Liver Failure after Taking 'Health Supplement,'" *NY Post*, January 3, 2020.

417   Holly Vogtman, "Dietary Supplement Use Reaches All Time High," *CRN USA*, September 30, 2019.

that they are simply excreted in your urine. That is some expensive pee! Some examples of water-soluble supplements are vitamin C (ascorbic acid) and all forms of vitamin B (thiamin, riboflavin, niacin, pantothenic acid, vitamin B6, biotin, folacin, and vitamin B12). These vitamins must be consumed regularly, because there is no storage form in the body (B12 being an exception). In fact, doctors prefer their patients to get these vitamins naturally from food, unless you are unable to get an adequate amount of a certain vitamin from your diet.

The supplement industry is thriving today because it capitalizes on our strong desires for good health. Isn't that why both myself and the woman who suffered from acute liver failure had experimented with them? Our intentions were pure, but it was our lack of education that led us in the wrong direction.

Broadly construed, just because a supplement claims to promote health does not necessarily mean it is healthy. I am going to illustrate how this relates to the following types of supplements: multivitamins, trace elements, sodium, magnesium, antioxidants, and fish oil.

MULTIVITAMINS

Growing up, my family always had multivitamins in our pantry. I never complained about having to take my vitamins. In fact, I looked forward to them. I remember one year my mom packed a handful of gummy vitamins when we went on vacation. A few days later, she had found the zip lock bag empty and discovered that my cousins had eaten them, assuming they were candy. My cousins quickly learned of their mistake when they started experiencing uncomfortable digestion pains. These vitamins taste so good that they are easily mistaken for candy due to their sugar content. You may be surprised that by learning more about the vitamins found in foods in our daily diet, we may not need to rely on expensive supplements that rarely accomplish what they claim.

TRACE ELEMENTS

Outside of sugar, commercial multivitamins usually contain a majority of the nine trace elements that are essential for cell function: chromium, copper, fluorine, iodine, iron, manganese, molybdenum, selenium, and zinc. Your body is unable to synthesize these trace elements, so it is essential to obtain them from your diet. Since we only need twenty milligrams a day, most people can consume the recommended amount of trace elements from their diet alone.[418] By taking a supplement with trace elements, you can easily surpass the twenty-milligram limit.

If you are exceeding consumption consistently, it can pose serious health concerns.[419] For example, excess zinc interferes with the absorption of iron and copper (all being

---

418   Sandra May, "Minerals (Lesson 8)," *LSU Agriculture Center,* February 25, 2019.

419   "Vitamins and Minerals," *Harvard Health: HelpGuide,* accessed February 1, 2021.

trace elements), and excess copper has been indicated in cirrhosis (irreversible late-stage liver damage). [420]

SODIUM

A surplus in any mineral (trace or not) has the potential to interact with other substances resulting in negative health effects. Minerals take on the main role of maintaining water balance throughout the body. Some minerals help regulate protein structure (including hair, nails, and skin), while other proteins are essential for healthy bones and muscles.[421] For instance, sodium is indispensable in supplying cellular stability, assisting in muscle and nerve function, and managing blood pressure.[422] Unfortunately, many people ingest excess sodium by adding it to their meals or eating prepackaged foods with large amounts of this mineral designed to enhance

---

420 J. K. Campbell and C. F. Mills, "Effects of Dietary Cadmium and Zinc on Rats Maintained on Diets Low in Copper," *The Proceedings of the Nutrition Society 33*, no. 1 (May 1974): 15A–16A; Committee on Diet and Health Food and Nutrition Board Commission on Life Sciences National Research Council, *Diet and Health: Implications for Reducing Chronic Disease Risk* (Washington DC: National Academies Press (US), 1989), 14 Trace Elements; National Research Council (US), *Copper in Drinking Water* (Washington DC: National Academies Press (US), 2000), 4 Disorders of Copper Homeostasis; National Research Council (US), *Copper in Drinking Water* (Washington DC: National Academies Press (US), 2000), 5 Health Effects of Excess Copper; A. N. Pandit and S. A. Bhave, "Copper and Indian Childhood Cirrhosis," *Indian Pediatrics 20*, no. 12 (December 1983): 893–899.

421 "Minerals," *Medline Plus*, last modified October 19, 2020.

422 Healthwise Staff, "Sodium (Na) in Blood," *Michigan Medicine*, last modified December 8, 2019.

flavor. Diets with excess sodium have contributed to many health issues, such as high blood pressure and obesity.[423]

FOR THE SCIENTIFIC READER:

We must realize that salt is not equivalent to sodium. Salt symbolizes sodium chloride, and one gram of sodium chloride is equivalent to 390 milligrams of sodium.[424] In a situation with an imbalance of sodium, the body will try and compensate by sending calcium to bind with the sodium that is in excess to excrete it. Yet, when the calcium is assigned this new task, it is excreted with the excess sodium.[425]

MAGNESIUM

Most people receive enough minerals in the foods they eat, except for magnesium. Recently, people have become increasingly concerned about magnesium deficiency. Research indicated that 75 percent of Americans do not obtain the recommended dietary magnesium levels.[426]

---

423 Yuan Ma et al., "High Salt Intake: Independent Risk Factor for Obesity," *Hypertension 66*, no. 4 (October 2015): 843–849; "Salt and Sodium," *Harvard Health*, accessed February 13, 2021.

424 "Salt: The Role of Potassium and Sodium in Your Diet," *Centers for Disease Control and Prevention*, last modified June 29, 2018.

425 "Vitamins and Minerals," *Harvard Health: HelpGuide*, accessed February 1, 2021.

426 Mary P. Guerrera et al., "Therapeutic Uses of Magnesium," *American Family Physician 80*, no. 2 (July 2009): 157-162; K. Alaimo et al., "Dietary Intake of Vitamins, Minerals, and Fiber of Persons Ages 2 Months and Over in the United States: Third National Health and Nutrition Examination Survey, Phase 1, 1988-91," *Advance Data 258*, (November 1994): 1-28.

The Recommended Dietary Allowance (RDA) advises the magnesium consumption to be around four hundred milligrams for adult men and around 310 milligrams for adult women.[427] Just like any other minerals, low levels of magnesium are unhealthy. Dr. Jon Stahlman, an allergy and immunology specialist on staff at Emory University, explained to me that most critically ill patients in the intensive care unit of a hospital often suffer from hypomagnesemia (magnesium deficiency) because the body can become rapidly depleted of this element when critically ill. Studies have shown hypomagnesemia is oftentimes concealed behind other electrolyte abnormalities in the critically ill that will not improve until the magnesium is replaced.[428] Fortunately, most healthy people are able to easily maintain normal magnesium levels by consuming magnesium-rich foods in their diet, such as pumpkin, spinach, soy milk, brown rice, nuts, and dark chocolate.[429]

If your doctor agrees that a magnesium supplement would be beneficial for you, the NIH recommends adults do not exceed a 350-milligram dietary supplement. The NIH additionally suggests finding a magnesium dietary supplement that is easier for the body to digest, such as magnesium

---

427 National Institutes of Health, *Dietary Reference Intakes for Calcium, Phosphorus, Magnesium, Vitamin D, and Fluoride* (Washington DC: National Academies Press, 1997).

428 Bent-Are Hansen and Oyvind Bruserud, "Hypomagnesemia in Critically Ill Patients," *Journal of Intensive Care 6*, no. 21 (March 2018).

429 "Magnesium Rich Food," *Cleveland Clinic*, last modified November 24, 2020.

aspartate, magnesium citrate, magnesium lactate, and magnesium chloride.[430]

It is important to consult a doctor if starting magnesium supplements, especially if you take phosphorus supplements as well. While phosphorus is necessary for the growth and formation of your teeth, bones, and other cells and tissues, excess phosphorus affects the body's potential to utilize additional minerals, such as magnesium. [431]

ANTIOXIDANTS

Antioxidant supplements are marketed to promote overall health. So why don't they work as anticipated? The answer is complicated. Scientific research does not reveal antioxidant supplements, such as vitamins A, C, E, and selenium, to favor disease prevention.[432] In 2002, the National Cancer Institute (NCI) collaborated with Brigham and Women's Hospital for the *Physician's Health Study II (PHS II)* to determine if antioxidants vitamins C and E reduced disease risks. The study concluded that neither vitamin C nor vitamin E decreased the risks of cardiovascular disease (heart attacks and strokes),

430 "Magnesium," *NIH: Office of Dietary Supplements*, last modified March 24, 2020.

431 "Phosphorus in Diet," *Medline Plus*, last modified January 5, 2021; "Vitamins and Minerals," *Harvard Health: HelpGuide*, accessed February 1, 2021; Robin Madell, "What Is Phosphorus and Why Is It Important?," *Healthline*, last modified July 31, 2020.

432 Robin Madell, "What Is Phosphorus and Why Is It Important?," *Healthline*, last modified July 31, 2020.

cancer, and/or cataracts.[433] Astonishingly, an association was reported between vitamin E supplements and increased risk of hemorrhagic strokes (a stroke derived from a bleed in the brain).[434] Additional scientific studies reported an increased risk of prostate cancer.[435]

For the Scientific Reader:

This may have to do with the composition of vitamin E and what is considered to be a vitamin E supplement itself. In nature, vitamin E exists in eight strands (alpha-, beta-, gamma-, and delta-tocopherol

---

433 John Michael Gaziano, "Physicians' Health Study II (PHS II)," *NIH: Clinical Trials*, last modified February 28, 2018; Howard D Sesso et al., "Vitamins E and C in the Prevention of Cardiovascular Disease in Men: The Physicians' Health Study II Randomized Controlled Trial," *JAMA 300*, no. 18 (November 2008): 2123-33; "Antioxidants: In Depth," *NIH: National Center for Complementary and Integrative Health*, last modified November 2013.

434 Howard D. Sesso et al., "Vitamins E and C in the Prevention of Cardiovascular Disease in Men: The Physicians' Health Study II Randomized Controlled Trial," *JAMA 300*, no. 18 (November 2008): 2123-33; John Michael Gaziano, "Physicians' Health Study II (PHS II)," *NIH: Clinical Trials*, last modified February 28, 2018.

435 John Michael Gaziano, "Physicians' Health Study II (PHS II)," *NIH: Clinical Trials*, last modified February 28, 2018; "Antioxidants: In Depth," *NIH: National Center for Complementary and Integrative Health*, last modified November 2013; Eric A Klein et al., "Vitamin E and the Risk of Prostate Cancer: The Selenium and Vitamin E Cancer Prevention Trial (SELECT)," *JAMA 306*, no. 14 (October 2011): 1549-1556.

and alpha-, beta-, gamma-, and delta-tocotrienol).[436] In foods, vitamin E consists of a combination with all of these eight strands. On the other hand, supplements of vitamin E routinely consist of only one of the eight strands. Containing all eight strands of vitamin E is not required to be considered vitamin E in supplemental form. Dr. Neal Barnard, who has led groundbreaking research studies on the effects of diet on the human body, reported the consumption of imbalanced vitamin E strands (which you would consume through supplementation) will reduce your absorption of all other strands.[437] Just because vitamin E supplements may be marketed as "natural," does not provide any indication that the supplement is indeed natural. While some supplements may live up to their "natural" label, it is important to understand that the FDA does not have the authority to regulate supplements before entering the market; therefore, misguided truths may lie in their labels.

Here are two examples of adverse reactions that can happen while taking vitamin E supplements:

Taking vitamin E supplements may decrease the effectiveness of vitamin K, which is critical for blood clotting. [438] If you are on any anticoagulant drugs ("blood thinner medications"), such as Coumadin (brand name for Warfarin), it

---

436 "Vitamin E," *NIH: Office of Dietary Supplements*, last modified July 31, 2020.

437 *Ted Talk*, Neal Barnard: Power Foods for the Brain," September 20, 2016, video, 17:00.

438 Mayo Clinic Staff, "Vitamin E," *Mayo Clinic*, November 13, 2020.

is recommended to take an equal amount of vitamin K as your prescription dose.[439] Dr. Jon Stahlman recommends, "if you ever need to reverse the effects of Coumadin, you can administer an injection of vitamin K or increase the amount of vitamin K in their diet as Coumadin blocks vitamin K metabolism." It is also important to note that vitamin E may have a direct adverse reaction with anticoagulant medications as it can promote bleeding. This can become very serious in individuals on Coumadin, since this medication prevents blood clotting.[440]

FISH OIL

Scientists observed better overall health, specifically, reduced levels of heart disease in a diet high in fatty fish: salmon, herring, sardines, cod, and more.[441] In an attempt to make the benefits of omega-3 fish oil more readily available, supplements were made in 1980.[442] By 2012, fish oil had become the new fad—the most popular natural product listed in the states.[443] Unfortunately, the promising scientific evidence of fish oil supplements was short-lived. Dr. Eric Rimm, a professor of nutrition and epidemiology at the Harvard T. H. Chan School of Public Health, discussed the issue of assuming fish oil supplements come with no risk. He advised middle-aged

439 "Vitamin K," *NIH: Office of Dietary Supplements*, last modified February 24, 2020.

440 Ibid.

441 Mayo Clinic Staff, "Omega-3 in Fish: How Eating Fish Helps Your Heart," *Mayo Clinic*, September 28, 2019.

442 "Should You Consider Taking a Fish Oil Supplements?," *Harvard Health*, December 2017.

443 Ibid.

people not to take fish oil supplements without physician recommendation.[444] Similar to vitamin E supplements, the interaction between fish oil and anticoagulant medications (e.g., Coumadin) can increase bleeding risks.[445] My grandpop had been on Coumadin for a prolonged time and bled frequently. I remember when we would be eating dinner and I would look across the table and notice blood dripping down his arm. I asked him what had happened, and he tried to explain that he did not know he was even bleeding, and he was just a little "leaky." At the time, I did not understand the science behind the side effects of taking anticoagulants. I recently asked my grandpop if he took fish oil while he was taking Coumadin. He had, and that might have contributed toward his spontaneous daily bleeding.

In my research on fish oil, I came across something very surprising. Polychlorinated biphenyls, otherwise known as PCBs, are industrial chemicals that were banned in 1979 due to their strong linkage to cancer. However, more recently, scientists detected trace levels of PCBs in some brands of fish oil supplements. While small amounts of PCBs (in the nanograms) have been found in these supplements, there is an argument for the consumers to be notified of any level (>0) of PCBs.[446]

---

444 Ibid.

445 Mee Young Hong et al., "Fish Oil Contaminated with Persistent Organic Pollutants Reduces Antioxidant Capacity and Induces Oxidative Stress without Affecting Its Capacity to Lower Lipid Concentrations and Systemic Inflammation in Rats," *The Journal of Nutrition* 145, no. 5 (May 2015): 939–44.

446 Andrew Weil, "PCBs in Fish Oil Supplements," *Dr Weil*, July 8, 2010.

Even with a high level of concern with fish oil supplements, many people continue to believe fish oil is right for them because they believe the benefits outweigh the associated risks. According to the American Heart Association, omega-3 fish oil supplements have potential beneficial outcomes in certain patient groups. Studies show they may aid in reducing the mortality from coronary heart disease by approximately 10 percent and they recommend reasonable supplementation under the direction of a physician.[447]

IF YOU DO TAKE FISH OILS, HAVE YOU EVER CONSIDERED ALGAE OIL?

Dr. Asha Subramamanian, a doctor of family medicine and a certified plant-based nutritionist, recommends using a plant-based omega-3 source like algae instead of fish oil.[448] People tend to forget that fish are a prime source of omega-3 fatty acids, because fish, like salmon, get their nutrients (including the omega-3 fatty acids) from eating algae.[449] Algae is the original source of these omega-3 acids. Algae oil absorbs and

---

447 David S. Siscovick et al., "Omega-3 Polyunsaturated Fatty Acid (Fish Oil) Supplementation and the Prevention of Clinical Cardiovascular Disease," *AHA Journal 135*, (April 2017): e867–e884.

448 *Plant Based News*, "Which Supplements Are Necessary? Doctors Weigh In," March 26, 2020, video, 5:19.

449 "Omega-3 Fatty Acids," *NIH: Office of Dietary Supplements*, last modified October 1, 2020; John L Harwood, "Algae: Critical Sources of Very Long-Chain Polyunsaturated Fatty Acids," *Biomolecules 9*, no. 11 (November 2019): 708; Bhakti Tanna and Avinash Mishra, "Metabolites Unravel Nutraceutical Potential of Edible Seaweeds: An Emerging Source of Functional Food," *Comprehensive Reviews in Food Science and Food Safety 17*, no. 6 (October 2018).

metabolizes like fish oil yet is also just as nutritious as cooked salmon. The same cannot be said for fish oil.[450] Compared to fish oil, algae oil is reported free from toxins, and it's more neutral flavor is associated with a decreased risk of digestion complications. [451, 452]

Anything that is not prescribed by your doctor, such as supplements, should still be addressed with your doctor.

JUST BECAUSE A SUPPLEMENT SAYS IT IS NATURAL DOES NOT MEAN IT IS SAFE.

Similar to the digestion of food, everyone may react differently to the digestion of supplements, especially if there is more than one medication being added to the body. Recently, I thought a lot about the safety of supplements versus prescribed medications. There are many more steps taken to ensure the safety and effectiveness of prescription medications. The Food and Drug Administration (FDA) is responsible for regulating drugs before they enter the market (pre-approval phase) and after entering the market (post-approval phase).[453] In addition to adhering to the professional

---

450   Linda M. Arterburn et al., "Algal-Oil Capsules and Cooked Salmon: Nutritionally Equivalent Sources of Docosahexaenoic Acid," *Journal of the American Dietetic Association 108*, no. 7 (2008): 1204–1209.

451   John L Harwood, "Algae: Critical Sources of Very Long-Chain Polyunsaturated Fatty Acids," *Biomolecules 9*, no. 11 (November 2019): 708.

452   Alan S. Ryan et al., "Clinical Overview of Algal-Docosahexaenoic Acid: Effects on Triglyceride Levels and Other Cardiovascular Risk Factors," *American Journal of Therapeutics 16*, no. 2 (March-April 2009): 183–192.

453   Agata Dabrowska and Susan Thaul, "How FDA Approves Drugs and Regulates Their Safety and Effectiveness," *Congressional Research Service*, May 8, 2018.

regulations, most Americans take even further steps of precaution to research the side effects, appropriate dosage, effectiveness, and noted precautions of their prescribed medications. Medications often come with stickers reminding you to "not take with alcohol" or to "take with food." There is no harm in taking extra precautions.

So, why are we not taking extra precautions before consuming supplements and researching what not to take with them? The risk of a pharmacokinetic (how the body metabolizer) interaction always exists.[454] If simultaneously consumed, the competition for metabolizing may produce a change in composition, reducing the effectiveness of one of the medications or, even worse, increasing the risk of a negative human health effect.[455] Dr. Su Sachar, a gastroenterologist affiliated with Northwestern Medicine Delnor Hospital Geneva, discussed the genetic susceptibility of supplemental reactions. She explained that some people have problems with their enzymes and liver that may cause issues in the way they metabolize supplements and others may run into issues with supplements causing an adverse effect on blood clotting.[456] Unfortunately, it is not just the interactions that people should be concerned with, it is the safety of the supplement itself. Supplements are constantly advertised on social media, television, blogs, and word of mouth. You can go to any local grocery store and find an aisle of supplements full of all different brands and types. The availability and

---

454 Gary N. Asher et al., "Common Herbal Dietary Supplement-Drug Interactions," *American Family Physician* 96, no. 2 (July 2017): 101–107.

455 Ibid.

456 *The Doctors*, "Woman Almost Dies After Taking Daily Supplements?," February 19, 2020, video, 4:50.

convenience of supplements make them seem safe. Would products that are unsafe be readily available to consumers? The simple, but unfortunate answer, is yes. "The U.S. Food and Drug Administration (FDA) does not have the authority to review dietary supplement products for safety and effectiveness before they are marketed."[457] Federal law does not require FDA regulation in the pre-approval phase of supplements. Due to the Dietary Supplement Health and Education Act of 1994, the FDA has the opportunity to regulate in the post-approval phase (check for products that are adulterated, misbranded, or just simply unsafe), but by this time, the supplement had already been available to the public.[458] As Harvard Health states, "Manufacturers can sell these without submitting evidence of their purity, potency, safety, efficacy."[459] The estimated fifty thousand US unreported adverse reactions due to supplementation each year has been referred to as "American Roulette" by Harvard's Dr. Peter Cohen.[460] The regulation for supplements is not the same as it is for prescription medications and people must understand this!

ARE SUPPLEMENTS RECOMMENDED TO TREAT OR PREVENT CORONAVIRUS?

Currently, the year is 2021 and we are amid the coronavirus pandemic. Now, more than ever, people are curious to know if there are any supplements they should take to boost their immune system. While the best way to promote immunity is

457 "What You Need to Know About Dietary Supplements," *FDA*, last modified November 29, 2017.

458 "Dietary Supplements." *FDA*, last modified August 16, 2019.

459 "Supplements: A Scorecard," *Harvard Health*, April 2012.

460 Ibid.

naturally through the intake of nutrient-dense foods (which include plentiful minerals and vitamins), certain populations may be at elevated risks of disease or deficiency and may benefit from a vitamin/mineral supplement. There is no known evidence that supplements may prevent, treat, or cure the coronavirus, but it is always a good idea to maintain a healthy, balanced diet and to ask for and/or follow your doctor's supplement recommendations if you fall into one of the at-risk populations for vitamin/mineral deficiencies. Do not fall for the trap of testimonials, especially from celebrities and politicians who claim that vitamin D supplements saved them during their COVID-19 experience. They are not a reliable source.

WHAT POPULATIONS MAY BENEFIT FROM TAKING SUPPLEMENTS?

Certain expert groups have identified individuals who would benefit from supplements. Vegetarians/vegans, pregnant women, and people who have low bone density are some populations that might benefit the most from taking supplements.

VEGETARIANS/VEGANS

The diet lifestyle of plant-based eaters can be very healthy; however, simply cutting out meat and poultry will not automatically provide you with a better quality-of-life. Certain proteins that are not permitted in a vegetarian and or vegan diet may lead to a nutrient deficiency if not accounted for. It is possible to achieve a very well-rounded nutritious diet without taking supplements; however, doctors may still recommend them.

VITAMIN B12

Naturally, vitamin B12 (Cobalamin) is mostly found in animal sources. While B12 can be found in nutritional yeast, certain mushrooms, and some fortified foods, obtaining adequate levels of B12 is definitely more of a challenge for plant-based eaters. Vitamin B12 deficiency can lead to a form of anemia.[461] Dr. Neal Barnard, along with general practitioner Dr. Vivian Chen and many other doctors, highly recommend vegans take a B12 supplement.[462] There are four different kinds of B12: Cyanocobalamin, Hydroxocobalamin, Methylcobalamin, and Adenosylcobalamin. Based on your genetics, diet, and lifestyle, one form of B12 may be more beneficial for you. The FDA has approved Cyanocobalamin B12 supplements, the well-known form, for vitamin B12 deficiency.[463] Crystallization characteristics of Cyanocobalamin, along with the ability to resist oxidation from the air, allows Cyanocobalamin to be utilized and to exist in some multivitamins.[464] However, it is still not entirely recommended to take them without a physician's approval.

For the Scientific Reader:

The inactive form of vitamin B12: Cyanocobalamin requires a cyanide molecule. Biochemically

461 "Vitamin B12," *NIH: Office of Dietary Supplements*, last modified January 15, 2021.

462 *Plant Based News*, "Which Supplements Are Necessary? Doctors Weigh In," March 26, 2020, video, 5:19.

463 National Center for Biotechnology Information, "Cyanocobalamin," *PubChem*, accessed February 1, 2021.

464 "Vitamin B12 (Cyanocobalamin)," *Medicine LibreText*, last modified August 14, 2020.

Cyanocobalamin avidly (accumulated affinities of non-covalent interactions) binds to cyanide (-CN) in the purification of activated charcoal. [465] Cyanide is not typically dangerous and is present in trace levels in foods.[466] However, energy is required to convert and/or remove cyanide, which could contribute to the glutathione reserve depletion that may occur in Cyanocobalamin detoxification.[467] If the glutathione reserve empties, cyanide toxicity may result from Cyanocobalamin, especially in people who suffer from renal (kidney) failure.[468]

B12 deficiencies are not always easy to identify. Plant-based diets are rich in Folacin (vitamin B9), also known as folate, which takes on a role in the production of red blood cells, similar to vitamin B12. Due to this B12 deficiency, symptoms may be hidden due to the high levels of Folacin; yet, increased Folacin cannot correct a B12 deficiency.[469] A deficiency in B12 can lead to hyperhomocysteinemia (high

465 Ibid; V. Herbert, "Vitamin B-12: Plant Sources, Requirements, and Assay," *The American Journal of Clinical Nutrition 48*, no. 3 (September 1988): 852–858.

466 Nadia Chaouali et al., "Potential Toxic Levels of Cyanide in Almonds (Prunus Amygdalus), Apricot Kernels (Prunus Armeniaca), and Almond Syrup," *ISRN Toxicology 2013*, (September 2013): 610648.

467 "Step 2 in MTHFR Support: How to Choose the Right B12 for You," *MTHRF Support Australia*, accessed February 1, 2021.

468 John David Spence, "B Vitamin Therapy for Homocysteine: Renal Function and Vitamin B12 Determine Cardiovascular Outcomes," *Clinical Chemistry and Laboratory Medicine 51*, no. 3 (March 2013): 633–637.

469 "Folate (Folic Acid) – Vitamin B9," *Harvard Health*, accessed February 1, 2021.

levels of homocysteines). B12 deficiency can also lead to a serious condition called pernicious anemia.[470]

For the Scientific Reader:

Homocysteines are found in everyone's blood and are non-proteinogenic amino acids, meaning they are not found in the genetics of organisms. Elevated levels may lead to arterial damage, including the entrance of blood clots in blood vessels, osteoporosis (bone-thinning disease), and CVD.[471] A simple blood test can determine your levels of homocysteines.

A B12 deficiency may also lead to reduced levels of antioxidants.[472] A key benefit to following a strict plant-based diet is the increased levels of antioxidants. When you see colorful, bright foods, the word "antioxidant" should scream at you because this is where most of them are found.[473]

---

470 Lydia Krause et al., "Pernicious Anemia," *Healthline*, May 13, 2020.

471 Kiara Anthony, "High Homocysteine Level (Hyperhomocysteinemia)," *Healthline*, last modified September 18, 2018; W. Herrmann et al., "Total Homocysteine, Vitamin B(12), and Total Antioxidant Status in Vegetarians," *Clinical Chemistry 47*, no. 6 (June 2001): 1094–1101; Filippo Brocadello et al., "Irreversible Subacute Sclerotic Combined Degeneration of the Spinal Cord in a Vegan Subject," *Nutrition 23*, no. 7-8 (July-August 2007): 622–624.

472 Tomohiro Bito et al., "Vitamin B12 Deficiency Results in Severe Oxidative Stress, Leading to Memory Retention Impairment in *Caenorhabditis Elegans*," *Redox Biology 11*, (April 2017): 21–29; Erik E. Van de Lagemaat et al., "Vitamin B12 in Relation to Oxidative Stress: A Systematic Review," *Nutrients 11*, no. 2 (February 2019): 482.

473 Justine Butler, "Essential Guide to Antioxidants on a Vegan Diet," *Plant Based News*, last modified October 1, 2020.

Unfortunately, if the missing nutrients from animals are not accounted for in a plant-based diet, the effects of a vitamin B12 deficiency will adversely affect the intended lifestyle of going vegetarian and/or vegan.

PREGNANT WOMEN

It is easy to assume pregnant women should take supplements, because not only do they have to provide for their own life, but they have to provide for the life of the baby living off of their nutrients. Similar to how there are well-known substances to avoid during pregnancy (such as foods high in mercury, cigarettes and, of course, alcohol), there are also substances less commonly known to avoid during pregnancy, including a variety of supplements. [474] As previously mentioned, antioxidant supplements are generally not recommended by medical professionals for the average person and tend to carry risks for a pregnant person. Vitamin A is fat-soluble, meaning it is not excreted in the urine, transported in lipoproteins, and, therefore, associated with an increased risk of toxicity. Certain vitamins, when accumulated in the body, may be toxic and result in harmful symptoms. While vitamin A is generally included in your typical prenatal vitamin, any additional supplement of it is strongly not recommended.

For the Scientific Reader:

The body will store excess vitamin A in the liver, since it is unable to excrete what it does not need. Due to this, liver damage may result, which can cause congenital

---

474 "Fetal Alcohol Spectrum Disorders (FASDs)," *Centers for Disease Control and Prevention*, last modified October 8, 2020.

birth abnormalities in children.[475] In addition to antioxidant supplements, some traditional Chinese medications (e.g., Dong Quai) and plants (e.g., black cohosh and goldenseal) are not advised for pregnant women. [476] If you are curious about a specific type, ask your doctor for professional advice.

While there is an increased list of precautions to take when caring for the baby and your nutritional needs, there is also an increased need for macro and micronutrients. The intake of macronutrients (proteins, fats, and carbohydrates) must significantly be increased to keep up the demand of creating life. While some can fulfill the significantly raised micronutrient requirements through the nutrients in their increased intake of macronutrients, most pregnant women tend to struggle with this, causing supplements to come in.[477] The American College of Obstetricians and Gynecologists (ACOG) advises pregnant women to utilize a prenatal vitamin supplement, along with an additional folic acid (B9)

475 Juliana Gutierrez-Mazariegos et al., "Vitamin A: A Multifunctional Tool for Development," *Seminars in Cell & Developmental Biology* 22, no. 6 (2011): 603–610; Sabina Bastos Maia et al., "Vitamin A and Pregnancy: A Narrative Review," *Nutrients* 11, no. 3 (March 2019): 681; Anthony R. Scialli, "Does Vitamin A Cause Birth Defects?," *Relias Media*, November 1, 2001.

476 Dena Westphalen, "Supplements During Pregnancy: What's Safe and What's Not," *Healthline*, last modified August 13, 2020; "Complementary and Alternative Medicine," St. Luke's Hospital, accessed February 1, 2021; "Dong Quai," *Medline Plus*, last modified January 29, 2021.

477 Alison D. Gernand et al., "Micronutrient Deficiencies in Pregnancy Worldwide: Health Effects and Prevention," *Nature Reviews Endocrinology* 12, no. 5 (June 2016): 274–289.

supplement.[478] Prenatal vitamins should be taken during pregnancy and breastfeeding and should be thought of as a highly recommended multivitamin targeted to meet the micronutrient needs for you and your baby. The use of prenatal vitamin supplements for pregnant women has shown outstanding health outcomes.[479] Prenatal vitamins allow pregnant women to reach their new recommended levels of iron, which is essential in the development and support of the placenta and the fetus, as it allows the body to create blood to supply oxygen to the fetus.[480] Prenatal vitamins are associated with a reduced risk of preeclampsia, a life-threatening pregnancy complication identified with high blood pressure, presence of proteins in the urine, blurred vision, headaches, and renal abnormalities.[481] Although most prenatal vitamins include folate, the CDC recommends all pregnant women consume at least four hundred mcg of folate (folic acid) each day.[482] Due to this additional folate, supplements may be ben-

478   "Nutrition During Pregnancy," *The American College of Obstetricians and Gynecologists*, June 2020.

479   Christina Oh et al., "Vitamin and Mineral Supplementation During Pregnancy and Maternal, Birth, Child Health and Development Outcomes in Low- and Middle- Income Countries: A Systematic Review and Meta-Analysis," *Nutrients 12*, no. 2 (2012): 491.

480   Mayo Clinic Staff, "Prenatal Vitamins: Why They Matter, How to Choose," *Mayo Clinic*, May 1, 2020.

481   Lisa M. Bodnar et al., "Periconceptional Multivitamin Use Reduces the Risk of Preeclampsia," *American Journal of Epidemiology 164*, no. 5 (September 2006): 470–477; Mayo Clinic Staff, "Preeclampsia," *Mayo Clinic*, March 19, 2020.

482   "Folic Acid," *Center for Disease Control and Prevention*, last modified April 11, 2018.

eficial. Research has shown folic acid supplements to reduce the risk of neural tube defects (e.g., spina bifida) up to 70 percent.[483] If you refer back to the gluten and grains chapter, you will notice that the FDA required the fortification of folic acid to all enriched grains. The positive health effects of folic acid are groundbreaking and should be taken very seriously. Pregnant women must receive plentiful amounts of folic acid utilizing food and supplementation. There is an increased need for additional micronutrients during pregnancy (e.g., iron, vitamin D, iodine, etc).[484] Most of these needs should be fulfilled from the prenatal vitamin; however, it is always a good idea to have a consultation with your primary care physician and/or OBGYN to create a schedule during this beautiful time.

VITAMIN D

Vitamin D is an exception to the game. It is hard to get vitamin D in your diet, and for this reason, vitamin D supplements may make sense for certain individuals. Vitamin D is often referred to as the "sunshine vitamin," because exposure to sunlight can biochemically produce vitamin D in our

---

483 "Folic Acid," *Spina Bifida Association*, accessed February 1, 2021.

484 Priya Soma-Pillay et al., "Physiological Changes in Pregnancy," *Cardiovascular Journal of Africa 27*, no. 2 (March-April 2016): 89–94; Bruce W. Hollis and Carol L. Wagner, "Nutritional Vitamin D Status During Pregnancy: Reasons for Concern," *CMAJ: Canadian Medical Association Journal 174*, no. 9 (April 2006): 1287-90; *Plant Based News*, "Which Supplements Are Necessary? Doctors Weigh In," March 26, 2020, video, 5:19.

bodies.[485] Sunlight is responsible for creating two forms of ultraviolet radiation: UVA and UVB. In this case, we want to focus on UVB, because it provides needed energy for the creation of vitamin D in your body.[486]

For the Scientific Reader:

For the body to make vitamin D, UVB will penetrate through the skin to convert cutaneous 7-dehydrocholesterol to the pre-vitamin D3, an intermediate in the production of vitamin D3.[487]

People can fulfill their vitamin D needs through vitamin D3 (cholecalciferol), as just stated, or vitamin D2 (ergocalciferol). Vitamin D2 is commonly human-made and added to specific foods, such as mushrooms.[488] Most dairy and non-dairy milks are fortified with vitamin D3.[489] Dietary supplements of vitamin D may exist in either form.

485 Rathish Nair and Arun Maseeh, "Vitamin D: The "Sunshine" Vitamin," *Journal of Pharmacology & Pharmacotherapeutics* 3, no. 2 (April-June 2012): 118–126; "Vitamin D," *NIH: Office of Dietary Supplements*, last modified on October 9, 2020.

486 "Vitamin D and Your Health: Breaking Old Rules, Raising New Hopes," *Harvard Health*, last modified May 17, 2019.

487 "Vitamin D," *NIH: Office of Dietary Supplements*, last modified October 9, 2020.

488 Glenn Cardwell et al., "A Review of Mushrooms as a Potential Source of Dietary Vitamin D," *Nutrients* 10, no. 10 (October 2018): 1498.

489 "Vitamin D for Milk and Milk Alternatives," *FDA*, January 4, 2018.

For the Scientific Reader:

The dietary supplement of vitamin D3 is produced through the ultraviolet irradiation of 7-dehydrocholesterol from lanolin ("wool yolk") and the cholesterol chemical conversion.[490] On the other hand, the dietary supplement of vitamin D2 is produced through the ultraviolet irradiation of ergosterol (a sterol in the cell membrane) in yeast.[491] Both vitamin D2 and vitamin D3 dietary supplements can raise the blood serum 25(OH)D.[492] However, there is evidence that vitamin D3 can increase the blood serum of 25(OH)D even more than vitamin D2.[493]

490 "Vitamin D," *NIH: Office of Dietary Supplements,* last modified October 9, 2020.

491 Ibid; Michael F. Holick, "Vitamin D Deficiency," *The New Journal of Medicine 357,* no. 3 (2007): 266–281.

492 John F. Aloia et al., "Vitamin D Intakes to Attain a Desired Serum 25-Hydroxyvitamin D Concentration," *The American Journal of Clinical Nutrition 87,* no. 6 (June 2008): 1952–1958.

493 Laura Tripkovic et al., "Comparison of Vitamin D2 and Vitamin D3 Supplementation in Raising Serum 25-Hydroxyvitamin D Status: A Systematic Review and Meta-Analysis," *The American Journal of Clinical Nutrition 95,* no. 6 (May 2012): 1357–1364; Laura Tripkovic et al., "Daily Supplementation with 15 μG Vitamin D2 Compared with Vitamin D3 to Increase Wintertime 25-Hydroxyvitamin D Status in Healthy South Asian and White European Women: A 12-Wk Randomized, Placebo-Controlled Food-Fortification Trial," *The American Journal of Clinical Nutrition 106,* no. 2 (2017): 481–490.

All vitamin D supplements have equal abilities to prevent rickets, a vitamin D deficiency that softens and weakens the bones of children. [494]

Direct sunlight exposure can carry out some of the vitamin D requirements in most people.[495] Vitamin D deficiency has been increasing internationally ever since the shift of work from the farm to the office.[496] Since exposure to sunlight accounts for 90 percent of the vitamin D production in the body, when people stepped out of the sunlight and into the artificial light, they brought vitamin D deficiencies with them. You cannot synthesize vitamin D from an office, even if the sun is shining through the windows, because UVB radiation cannot penetrate glass.[497] An estimated 70 percent of Americans lack adequate levels of vitamin D.[498]

There are many factors to account for when assessing your needs for vitamin D supplements. Regarding sunlight exposure itself, you must think about the seasons, time and length of the day, weather (sunny or cloudy), and air quality (clear

494 Mariana Costa Silva and Tania Weber Furlanetto, "Intestinal Absorption of Vitamin D: A Systematic Review," *Nutrition Reviews 76*, no. 1 (2018): 60–76; Mayo Clinic Staff, "Rickets," *Mayo Clinic*, May 14, 2019.

495 Institute of Medicine, *Dietary Reference Intakes for Calcium and Vitamin D* (Washington DC: National Academy Press, 2011).

496 Harin Jeong et al., "Vitamin D Status and Associated Occupational Factors in Korean Wage Workers: Data from the 5th Korea National Health and Nutrition Examination Survey (KNHANES 2010–2012)," *Annals of Occupational and Environmental Medicine 26*, no. 28 (September 2014).

497 Arash Hossein-Nezhad and Michael F Holick, "Vitamin D for Health: A Global Perspective," *Mayo Clinic Proceedings 88*, no. 7 (June 2013): 720–755.

498 "Supplements: A Scorecard," *Harvard Health*, April 2012.

or smog).[499] Not only would your vitamin D levels differ depending on where you live, but they also depend on your skin color. People of color may have issues with lower circulating vitamin D levels, since they possess a larger amount of melanin, a pigment in the epidermal skin layer responsible for the biological functions of skin and hair pigmentation, photo-protection of the skin and eyes, and vitamin D synthesis. [500] Older people are also at a higher risk of vitamin D deficiencies.[501]

For the Scientific Reader

People of color on average have decreased blood serum 25(OH)D levels compared to Caucasians.[502]

---

499 "Vitamin D," *NIH: Office of Dietary Supplements*, last modified October 9, 2020.

500 Minela Aida Maranduca et al., "Synthesis and Physiological Implication of Melanic Pigments," *Oncology Letters 17*, no. 5 (February 2019): 4183–4187; Angel Fernandez-Flores et al., "Histopathology of Aging of the Hair Follicle," *Journal of Cutaneous Pathway 46*, no. 7 (July 2019): 508–519; Michela Starace et al., "Use of Nail Dermoscopy in the Management of Melanonychia: Review," *Dermatology Practical & Conceptual 9*, no. 1 (January 2019): 38–43; "Vitamin D," *NIH: Office of Dietary Supplements*, last modified October 9, 2020; National Institutes of Health, *Dietary Reference Intakes for Calcium, Phosphorus, Magnesium, Vitamin D, and Fluoride* (Washington DC: National Academies Press, 1997).

501 Institute of Medicine, *Dietary Reference Intakes for Calcium and Vitamin D* (Washington DC: National Academy Press, 2011).

502 LaVerne L. Brown et al., "The Vitamin D Paradox in Black Americans: A Systems-Based Approach to Investigating Clinical Practice, Research, and Public Health - Expert Panel Meeting Report," *BMC Proceedings 12*, no. 6 (2018).

The National Institutes of Health recommends around six hundred IU (international units)/fifteen mcg of vitamin D daily.[503] You can assess your vitamin D levels through a blood test. You want to make sure your vitamin D levels are over thirty nanograms per milliliter.[504] If they are under, consult with your doctor about the possibility of starting vitamin D supplements.

On the FDA website, you can find the statement, "Unlike drugs, supplements are not permitted to be marketed for the purpose of treating, diagnosing, preventing, or curing diseases."[505] Supplements which claim to "lower weight," "cure acne," and "prevent heart disease" are not legitimate and a certain level of suspicion should be taken into account. People must stop looking for a quick fix for all of their health desires. Dr. Monique Tello, physician at Massachusetts General Hospital, author, and clinical instructor at Harvard Medical School, states, "The bottom line is that there is absolutely no substitute for a well-balanced diet, which is the ideal source of the vitamins and minerals we need."[506] Overall, supplements are not a good idea unless you fit into one of the exceptions: you follow a plant-based diet, you are pregnant, you have a vitamin deficiency, you have a specific type of disease that requires it, and/or your doctor has

503 "Vitamin D," *NIH: Office of Dietary Supplements*, last modified October 9, 2020.

504 Monique Tello, "Vitamin D: What's the "Right" Level?," *Harvard Health*, last modified April 16, 2020.

505 "What You Need to Know About Dietary Supplements," *FDA*, last modified November 29, 2017.

506 Monique Tello, "What Patients- and Doctors- Need to Know About Vitamins and Supplements," *Harvard Health*, March 16, 2018.

recommended it to you. However, if you are advised to take a supplement, do your research before buying the prettiest bottle or the brand that your favorite celebrity endorsed. Not all supplements are equal. Look for a supplement that has been tested by independent labs.[507] If you are buying your supplements online, it is a good idea to use non-commercial sites, such as the NIH or FDA, to fact check.[508] We want to consume our nutrients through our food and not through supplements, if possible. Maybe one day our culture will get there, but, as of now, remember if it is too good to be true, it probably is. Magic pills do not exist.

---

507 Ibid.

508 Ibid.

THREE

HOW TO OPTIMIZE YOUR EATING SCHEDULE

EIGHT

BREAKFAST

I was raised on the idea that "breakfast is the most important meal of the day." My parents always made sure we ate
breakfast before leaving for school. My brother Sam and I
always looked forward to the weekend, not because we did
not have to go to school, but because we got to indulge in
my dad's special breakfast of challah or brioche cinnamon
French toast—our favorite! Our friends made sure to sleep
over the night before to get in on the action, too. Breakfast
has always been my favorite meal of the day, and while my
breakfast meals look a lot different now than they did growing up, I have always prioritized and incorporated them into
my routine.

This is not the case for everyone. My mom and I have
always been morning people, yet I noticed when I moved
home during the COVID-19 pandemic, we suddenly had different eating routines. I typically eat my first meal an hour
after waking up; however, my mom will go for hours until
she has her first bite of food for the day because she practices intermittent fasting. I was surprised that she changed
and began questioning "who was right?" How much truth is
behind the belief that "breakfast is the most important meal

of the day"? Maybe I was wrong. Could my mom really be healthier by skipping breakfast?

MEDICAL MYTHOLOGY

Cereal makers have solidified the idea of a "healthy breakfast." In 1898, the Kellogg brothers revolutionized breakfast by inventing ready-to-go cereal, such as corn flakes.[509] The Kellogg brothers claimed their family business was for "biologic living," and that their cereals were to serve the purpose of indigestion helpers, therefore, making them beneficial to the body.[510] In 1917, John Harvey, one of the brothers, was quoted in *Good Health* magazine, stating, "In many ways, breakfast is the most important meal of the day."[511] Did cereal makers sell us a breakfast myth?

Similar to the theme with most nutritional upbringings, the Kellogg brothers were not the first people to come up with the idea of breakfast cereal. In 1863, Dr. James Caleb Jackson created Granula as the first cold cereal to serve the purpose of potentially curing different health ailments.[512] Unfortunately, with no previous cereals for inspiration, Granula struggled to obtain popularity because of its unappetizing appearance and tough texture.[513] Dr. Jackson became one of the biggest inspirations to the Kellogg brothers. John Harvey, himself, created one of the first popular American cereals, Grape-Nuts. This

509   Sarah Pruitt, "How an Accidental Invention Changed What Americans Eat for Breakfast?," *History*, last modified August 5, 2019.

510   Ibid.

511   Troy Lennon, "How the Kellogg Brothers Influenced the way Westerners Eat Breakfast," *Daily Telegraph*, August 8, 2018.

512   "Oldest Cereals Ever Created," *Oldest*, accessed January 30, 2021.

513   Ibid.

mixed grain cereal was made with whole-grain wheat flour, malted barley flour, salt, and dried yeast.[514] It was promoted to yield a perfect complexion for women's skin.[515] Grape-Nuts was described as a food with medicinal qualities that could lead a "straight road to health and comfort."[516] Ladies and gentlemen, drop everything. John Harvey Kellogg has done it. Grape-Nuts are the solution to everything. The labels and advertisements of Grape-Nuts are promising they solved all of our health issues. Were Grape-Nuts the only serious promising medicinal help? What were the social mores of the time that would make consumers want to believe this? Are Grape-Nuts really going to cure diseases?

You, the reader, are already ahead of the game here. In the Rise of Nutrition chapter, I discussed a brief timeline of FDA regulations for a uniform nutrition label. In the age of the Kellogg brothers, these regulations were not in place and companies could freely spew health claims. However, I am impressed that these companies attempted to conduct experimental studies, despite the paucity of business regulation.

Special K, one of Kellogg's most famous cereals, comes in fifteen different variations. The Special K Challenge is a two-week program for short-term weight loss that requires its participants to replace two meals a day with their low-calorie cereal meals.[517] The challenge was deemed effective and resulted in healthy overweight participants experiencing a significant reduction in body weight and waist circumference.

---

514 "Grape-Nuts," *Mr. Breakfast*, accessed January 30, 2021.

515 Ibid.

516 Ibid.

517 Kathleen M. Zelman, "The Special K Challenge," *WebMD*, accessed January 30, 2021.

As I scrolled through the study, I instantly noticed the small print in the middle of the article: "Funded by Kellogg."[518]

Just because the results from the study are truthful, does not mean they are accurate. In this case, Kellogg is telling the consumers to highly restrict their caloric intake. Of course they would see an immediate result! Also, there are other potential sources of bias, such as the failure to disclose the exercise patterns of participants. Kellogg was not the only breakfast company to hop on this bandwagon. Similar studies were conducted by Quaker Oats. These studies often testified that skipping breakfast was associated with significant health costs.

All of these studies made me more confused. Is breakfast really the most important meal of the day, or did breakfast makers trick us into believing this? The answer remains unclear from most of the case studies. What do doctors think about this? Christy C. Tangney, a clinical dietitian at Rush University Medical Center, has shared her expert opinion on many different platforms.[519] Although Kellogg and Quaker Oats may use the breakfast campaign to help advertise their brands, breakfast still may be beneficial.

If you think about it, when you are asleep, your body is in the longest period of fasting, and breakfast is literally set up to "break" your "fast." The myth is that when you eat breakfast you are able to "kick start" your metabolism. However, research has shown us that this is not true! Within a sixteen-week study to test the effect of breakfast on "kick

518   P Shaw et al., "The Effects of the Special K Challenge on Body Composition and Biomarkers of Metabolic Health in Healthy Adults," *Journal of Nutrition and Health Sciences* 2, no. 4 (November 2015).

519   "Why You Should Eat Breakfast," *Rush Edu*, accessed January 30, 2021.

starting" metabolisms, regardless if breakfast was eaten or not, the number of calories burned was not related.[520]

Besides the metabolism myth, there are many benefits to breakfast. Studies have shown breakfast to have a positive association with memory, concentration, cholesterol, diabetes, heart disease, and student performance.[521] When breakfast is skipped, your blood sugar is lowered, which may cause you to feel tired, and you may have diminished mental alertness. The only exception to blood sugar issues when skipping breakfast apply to fat adaptive intermittent fasters. It takes around two to four weeks to adjust to an intermittent fasting lifestyle. When fully accustomed to the patterned eating schedule, you are considered to be "fat adapted" and can effectively convert fatty acids and ketones into energy. Since I am not fat adapted and, therefore, not metabolically flexible, every time I skip breakfast, I feel like I need to take a nap. I feel weak and grumpy. I now realize that my mom does not feel "weak and grumpy" when skipping breakfast because she is "fat adapted" and, therefore, does not experience bad-tempered and sickly side effects.

For the Scientific Reader:
Once a person's body is fat adapted, they can easily shift from fueling on glucose, to glycogen, to fueling on fat. Individuals who are fat adapted are able to be

---

520 James A. Betts et al., "The Causal Role of Breakfast in Energy Balance and Health: A Randomized Controlled Trial in Lean Adults," *The American Journal of Clinical Nutrition 100*, no. 2 (August 2014): 539–547.

521 Antonio Affinita et al., "Breakfast: A Multidisciplinary Approach," *Italian Journal of Pediatrics 39*, no. 44 (July 2013); "Skipping Breakfast May Increase Coronary Heart Disease Risk," *Harvard Health*, July 23, 2013.

fueled by their own body fat, which is a consistent fuel source, providing them with more clarity. Refer back to our discussion with the ketogenic diet in the Fats chapter. Running on fats may improve brain health as a major ketone and beta-hydroxybutyrate (BHB) provides more energy per unit of oxygen used.[522]

It is well known that the human body follows a circadian rhythm, such as the sleep-wake cycle we tend to follow. However, this rhythm is typically thought of as just one cycle. Dr. Satchidananda Panda, professor and researcher at the Salk Institute in San Diego, acknowledged that not only is there a circadian clock of the body, but each organ runs on its own circadian clock.[523] The circadian cycle's original purpose is to create a schedule of eating when the sun is up and fasting when the sun is down. Since we are not nocturnal creatures, the light bulb's appearance over one hundred years ago has disrupted this natural cycle. Societal norms have altered our lifestyle, which has made it a rare occasion to find someone who does not eat when the sun is down. However, our bodies were not made to be fed constantly. Patterned eating is as ancient as the first humans.

I had the honor of chatting with Laurie Lewis, a certified intermittent fasting coach, who has changed the lives of thousands by explaining her research on intermittent fasting to create personal plans for individuals. Laurie made her way to the world of intermittent fasting after she struggled with stubborn hormonal fat, which appeared unmanageable with

522 Shelly Fan, "The Fat-Fueled Brain: Unnatural or Advantageous?," *Scientific American* (blog), October 1, 2013.

523 "Satchidananda Panda," *Salk Edu*, accessed January 30, 2021.

traditional remedies. After four-and-a-half years, she stumbled across a video on intermittent fasting that inspired her to begin experimenting the next day. The idea of a fasting lifestyle originally seemed foreign to her, since people tend to forget that our bodies were never made to eat all the time.

Emerging research has shown us that intermittent fasting may do more than just help an individual lose weight. Harvard Health details that "fasting is evolutionarily embedded within our physiology."[524]

Laurie explained how when her body adjusted to a clean fast, she was allowing her hormones to do their job correctly. There is a specific reason why she emphasized having a "clean" fast and not just a fast. There is a big difference between not eating anything for an extended period of time, fasting, and sneaking in one bite of food. It is human nature to believe eating only one bite of food within an extended period of time can be considered fasting; however, the biochemistry within your body will disagree. When you take that one bite of food, you trick your body into believing that you will be eating. If you try intermittent fasting, it is vital to avoid this. In a clean fast, all nutrients are to be avoided. Even one bite of food will throw the system off. However, you are allowed to consume unflavored water and black coffee. Besides that, all nutrients should be saved for consumption during your eating window when the body is in repair mode.

"The clean fast makes fasting easier and also puts the body into a state of repair —digestive, hormonal, and metabolic

---

524 Monique Tello, "Intermittent Fasting: Surprising Update," *Harvard Health*, June 29, 2018.

rest. If a person is skipping breakfast, they aren't fasting if they have flavors or nutrients, including coffee sweeteners or cream, lemon in water, zero-calorie sodas or flavored waters. Having those drinks while fasting ensures they are keeping insulin high and storing fat."

- LAURIE LEWIS.

In a fasted state, Laurie was able to hear her hormones trying to communicate with her. As previously discussed, the idea of allowing food to heal is an individual process, which is why it is important to stay in tune with your body. When your body is missing that fasted state, your hormones may be too busy to stop and communicate accurately with you. Once again, this process takes time. Listening to your body after one day of fasting will not be much help either. If you have ever fasted for one day or observed Yom Kippur (a Jewish holiday of atonement that requires fasting), I am sure you can relate when I say your body is going to point to signs for you to eat that cupcake. Your body will crave sugar, especially if it is used to eating sugar. You must be patient and allow your body to adjust to the foundation of fasting, adjust to become "fat adapted." Let the loud voices of sugar quiet down, so you can hear what your body is actually trying to tell you. You will notice your body start to crave the foods that nourish you and stray away from the foods that make you feel tired. I encourage you to check out Gin Stephen's book, *Fast. Feast. Repeat.*, which helped inspire Laurie.[525] This book is full of scientific research on the benefits of using a daily fasting regimen.

---

525   Gin Stephen, *Fast. Feast. Repeat.* (New York: St. Martin's Press, 2020).

For the Scientific Reader:

Hormones have independent jobs they are assigned to do; however, they sometimes become dependent on each other to fulfill these roles. This network of communication between hormones (such as cortisol, melatonin, estrogen, progesterone, insulin, ghrelin, and leptin) can work together in your favor, but not if they are unbalanced. Hormone balance is vital for optimizing your health. Most people in today's society have high insulin levels, preventing the body from tapping into its own fat storage. Therefore, high insulin is going to increase the amount of fat stored. This explains unhealthy blood sugar levels and contributes to an individual becoming pre-diabetic and diabetic. Intermittent fasting has been shown to restore this relationship with insulin and decrease insulin resistance, which is not only associated with a reduced risk of type II diabetes and fertility conditions like PCOS, but the regulation of insulin also seems to set the stage for other hormones to follow. The human growth hormone (HGH) is typically not reported when you are eating. HGH works to help your body repair your muscles and burn fat in the process. Intermittent fasting has shown an increase of HGH by 1,000 to 2,000 percent, since it is produced in a fasted state.[526] Dr. Satchidananda Panda studied the effects of intermittent fasting in mice, and the study found that those who followed time-restrictive eating were slimmer and healthier

526 Horne et al., "Study Finds Routine Periodic Fasting is Good for Your Health, and Your Heart," *Intermountain Medical Center*, April 3, 2011.

than the mice who did not follow an intermittent eating pattern. Both groups of mice consumed the same number of calories.[527]

Sleeping and fasting are both thought to make a difference in repairing our bodies. They both are patterns of food availability. Like sleep, the human body needs a pause. Fasting is the only other conscious effort we can do to put our bodies in a state of repair.

"Fasting, like sleep, isn't a 'thing.' It's imperative, and we can customize when and how long we fast and eat."

- LAURIE LEWIS.

The field of intermittent fasting is bigger than ever before. Science is continuing to expand our knowledge in the field as different studies have already found benefits of intermittent fasting, including an improved metabolism, lowered blood sugar, and decreased inflammation (which can ultimately help with issues ranging from improving asthma symptoms to lowering the risk of cancer by clearing out toxins).[528] Dr. Mark Mattson highlights the improvements in physical and mental health due to scheduled eating in an intermittent

527 "Satchidananda Panda," *Salk Edu*, accessed January 30, 2021.

528 Monique Tello, "Intermittent Fasting: Surprising Update," *Harvard Health*, June 29, 2018.

fasting lifestyle in a 2019 *New England Journal of Medicine Review.*[529]

Intermittent fasting allowed Laurie to finally lose her stubborn fat and feel more confident. However, it is important to note that intermittent fasting does not mean to just fast. Your body relies on food for survival. If you are fasting for periods that are too long for your body, or you are not eating enough calories in your eating window, it can be harmful for your body. It is important to consult a doctor or health coach, such as Laurie Lewis, if you decide to embark on this journey and find the right method for you (in general, intermittent fasting will include different eating windows and hours, depending on the person). Every human (except for pregnant or breastfeeding women) can eat in a pattern of time to extend their lives. Even people with type I diabetes can manage their insulin levels and get the metabolic and deep cellular healing that a daily fasting regimen provides. In today's food-centric world, it is hard to comply with the intermittent fasting lifestyle, especially because it does take time to adjust and become "fat adaptive." Dr. Satchidananda Panda and Dr. Valter Longo have proven that a 12:12 fasting:eating schedule not only will make you feel better within a week, but will increase the longevity of your life.[530]

---

529 Rafael de Cabo and Mark P. Mattson, "Effects of Intermittent Fasting on Health, Aging, and Disease," *The New England Journal of Medicine 381*, no. 26 (December 2019): 2541–2551.

530 Valter D. Longo and Satchindananda Panda, "Fasting, Circadian Rhythms, and Time Restricted Feeding in Healthy Lifespan," *Cell Metabolism 23*, no. 6 (2016): 1048–1059.

Tips from Laurie: Recap on how to become an intermittent faster:

- Eating in a pattern of time, even 12:12, has proven to increase lifespan.
- Having a fasting:eating pattern is the way human bodies were designed.
- The body needs metabolic, digestive, and hormonal healing as much as we need sleep.
- Fasting "clean" with plain, unflavored water and plain, black coffee (if you choose to have coffee).
- Fast clean and eat in an eating window.
- Saving all nutrients and flavors for the eating window allows each cell in the body to repair (autophagy).
- Having one to three meals in the eating window of your choice helps a person ward off disease and feel better.
- Do not diet or have a calorie-restricted diet. Eating well to satisfy the body's nutrient needs, coupled with fat-burning and ketosis, keeps the metabolic rate high.
- Choosing to eat in an eating window IS for all bodies and can be customized for each person's needs.
- Compliance is a different issue than whether it's an important, sustainable, and healthful practice. It is for everybody.

Once again, similar to saturated fats, science has confused us. Is breakfast the most important meal of the day? Who was right? While my mom skipping breakfast is definitely healthier than my dad's famous French toast, that does not mean it is healthier than my breakfast of avocado toast with eggs in the morning. I guess we could call it a tie. Breakfast companies have solidified this myth into our brains. There is nothing more "special" about breakfast than there is about dinner. The decision to become a breakfast eater or not should be decided based on your circumstances. Instead of focusing on when to "break the fast," we should focus on our eating schedule as a whole. Maybe not for the same reasons as one would today, but our ancestors ate on a time-restraint schedule. This idea got lost in translation through time and intermittent fasting is finally returning us to our roots. However, it is important to keep in mind that intermittent fasting does not discourage breakfast. If you follow an intermittent fasting lifestyle, do not feel like you must skip breakfast; experiment and find the right eating window for you.

NINE

DESSERT

___

"Life is uncertain, eat dessert first."

- ERNESTINE ULMER

Symbolically, this quote is made to teach the lesson of uncertainty and the importance of prioritizing what is important, such as your happiness in life. Dessert can put you in a good mood, contributing to your happiness. For example, chocolate is the most widely craved food.[531] Desserts, like chocolate, make you happy, because they stimulate the brain to release endorphins, chemicals in the body to relieve pain and stress, which can allow you to enter a state of euphoria.[532] Since we cannot predict the future and life is uncertain, why not eat your dessert first?

___

531 University of Bristol, "Chocolate Is the Most Widely Craved Food, but Is It Really Addictive?," *ScienceDaily*, September 12, 2007.

532 Astrid Nehlig, The Neuroprotective Effects of Cocoa Flavanol and its Influence on Cognitive Performance," *British Journal of Clinical Pharmacology 75*, no. 3 (March 2013): 716–27.

Unfortunately, the average person does not practice this saying. It is commonly instilled in our brains to not indulge in sweet and sugary foods before getting an adequate source of nutrients from dinner. Who made up this rule? Is it actually unhealthy to eat dessert before dinner?

Research has led us to believe that maybe we should take Ernestine's quote not just figuratively, but literally, as well. Eating any foods, especially sugary ones, close to your bedtime, may cause adverse health outcomes.

Refer back to the breakfast chapter, where I mentioned sleeping and fasting are the only two actions you can do to put your body in a state of repair. When you eat within two to three hours before you go to sleep, you are forcing your body to overwork and not allowing it the proper rest for your digestive system. Dr. Marvin Singh, internist and gastroenterologist, suggests to "avoid eating two to three hours before you go to bed." He emphasizes the importance of allowing the digestive system time to rest, so it can properly "clear up to reset for the next day."

NIGHT EATER SYNDROME

One in every ten obese individuals is affected by Night Eating Syndrome (NES), an eating disorder characterized by a delay in the circadian rhythm (the body's natural sleep-wake cycle) for the intake of food.[533] People with NES will consume at least 25 percent of their total daily calories after

---

533   "What Is Night Eating Syndrome?," *WebMD*, accessed February 15, 2021.

dinner, often including during nocturnal awakening to eat.[534] Many individuals who suffer from NES will also experience an absence of appetite in the morning (morning anorexia) and insomnia.[535] Regardless if you suffer from NES or not, consistently eating right before bedtime will result in similar symptoms. It takes around four to five hours for the stomach to completely empty.[536] Restarting the digestive process when you go to sleep (even if you are so tired that you can pass out), forces your digestive system to overwork. Imagine working a nine-to-five job, and then your boss makes you work overtime. This may tear at your emotional and physical health, since you are already exhausted and will have to exert more energy. This is very similar to how the digestive system feels, except it is never given a break at all, even after overtime hours.

For the Scientific Reader:
NES is attributed to a delay in the circadian rhythm. Excess nightly eating causes morning anorexia, which results in lower ghrelin levels in the morning compared to those without NES. Ghrelin is the hormone you should think of when your stomach starts to rumble. This hormone signals the brain to seek out food.

---

534 Healthwise Staff, "Night Eating Syndrome," *Michigan Medicine*, May 28, 2019; Kelly C. Allison and Ellen Tarves, "Treatment of Night Eating Syndrome," *The Psychiatric Clinic of North America 34*, no.4 (September 2011): 785–96.

535 Kelly C. Allison and Ellen Tarves, "Treatment of Night Eating Syndrome," *The Psychiatric Clinic of North America 34*, no.4 (September 2011): 785–96.

536 Richard Bowen, "Gastrointestinal Transit: How Long Does It Take?," *VIVO Pathophysiology*, accessed February 14, 2021.

Ghrelin has proven to be an effective hormone in regulating the circadian rhythm.[537] It is no surprise that insomnia is a side effect of NES since ghrelin levels increase as a factor of sleep deprivation.[538]

INSOMNIA

One of the first questions a doctor should ask if you struggle with insomnia is, "Do you eat dessert before you go to bed?" Sugar reduces sleep quality already regardless of what time of the day it is consumed, and eating sugar too close to bedtime can exacerbate those effects.[539]

As you may recall from the Inflammation chapter, sugar causes inflammation, and inflammation is associated with the presence of cytokines. Elevated cytokine levels have been linked to insomnia.[540]

Dr. Mark Hyman, a family physician and internationally known leader for functional medicine, leads a health revolution to support energy, happiness, longevity and using food as medicine. "Your brain chemistry and

537   Paola C. Yanninelli et al., "Ghrelin Effects on the Circadian System of Mice," *The Journal of Neuroscience: The Office Journal of the Society for Neuroscience 27*, no. 11 (March 2007): 2890–2895.

538   Sharad Taheri et al., "Short Sleep Duration is Associated with Reduced Leptin, Elevated Ghrelin, and Increased Body Mass Index," *PLoS Medicine 1*, no. 3 (December 2004): e62.

539   Marie-Pierre St-Onge et al., "Fiber and Saturated Fat are Associated with Sleep Arousals and Slow Wave Sleep," *Journal of Clinical Sleep Medicine 12*, no. 1 (January 2016): 19–24.

540   James M. Krueger, "The Role of Cytokines in Sleep Regulation," *Current Pharmaceutical Design 14*, no. 32 (2008): 3408–16.

hormones are controlled by what you eat and learning how to eat in a way that regulates those things is really key so that your energy is even." Dessert foods high in sugar tend to lower the production of serotonin and lower serotonin levels prompt sugar cravings.[541] Yet another vicious cycle thanks to sugar.

Serotonin is the precursor of melatonin.[542] Decreased serotonin, therefore, is associated with decreased melatonin. The brain produces melatonin as a response to the darkness outside, which helps to keep your body in line with its circadian rhythm, the natural sleep-wake cycle.[543] Melatonin has an inverse relationship with the hormone, cortisol. As melatonin levels increase in the evening, cortisol levels decrease and vice versa in the morning.

Serotonin deficiency is directly associated with sleeplessness and poor sleep onset. The relationship between serotonin and sleep is complicated, but overall, it is considered to help sleep, simply due to the fact that it is needed to produce melatonin.[544] When serotonin levels are thrown off, the quality and quantity of rapid eye movement (REM) sleep can be

541 Qurrat-ul-Aen Inam et al., "Effects of Sugar Rich Diet on the Brain Serotonin, Hyperphagia and Anxiety in Animal Model of Both Genders," *Pakistan Journal of Pharmaceutical Sciences* 29, no. 3 (2016): 757–763.

542 Richard Bowen, "The Pineal Gland and Melatonin," *VIVO Pathophysiology*, last modified November 2018.

543 "Melatonin: What You Need to Know," *NIH*, Last modified October 2019.

544 Carly Vandergriendt, "What's the Difference Between Dopamine and Serotonin?," *Healthline*, last modified July 16, 2020.

affected.[545] Sugar's impact on dopamine levels can further affect sleep quality. Similar to cocaine, sugar increases dopamine levels, which cause you to increase your alertness and stay awake.[546]

For the Scientific Reader:

Do not get confused between serotonin and dopamine. In the Inflammation chapter, I discussed how sugar becomes addicting, and the major reason is due to the increased dopamine production. Dopamine is associated with feelings of pleasure and is responsible for the activation of the rewards system within your brain that occurs when you eat sugar, making you crave it more. Serotonin is your happy hormone. It is possible to have high levels of dopamine, but low levels of serotonin; they are not the same.

Insomnia may be a symptom of magnesium deficiency.[547] As discussed in the supplements chapter, magnesium is one of the most challenging minerals to obtain and is one of the first levels to drop when sick. Magnesium deficiency can be

---

545   Reidun Ursin, "Serotonin and Sleep," *Sleep Medicine Reviews* 6, no. 1 (2002): 57-69; Edward F. Pace-Schott, "Serotonin and Dreaming," *Serotonin and Sleep: Molecular, Functional and Clinical Aspects* (2008): 307–324; "REM Sleep and Our Dreaming Lives," *S+ ResMed*, accessed February 15, 2021.

546   Nora D. Volkow et al., "Evidence That Sleep Deprivation Downregulates Dopamine d2r in Ventral Striatum in the Human Brain," *The Journal of Neuroscience* 32, no. 19 (May 2012): 6711–6717.

547   Michael J. Breus, "Magnesium – How it Affects Your Sleep," *Psychology Today (blog)*, May 2, 2018.

hard to identify, because it can be covered up by symptoms associated with other illnesses. Increasing your magnesium consumption by eating foods like pumpkin seeds, almonds, and spinach may aid in better sleep.[548]

So the next time that you have trouble sleeping, try to recall if you ate a sugary dessert before going to bed, specifically chocolate.

The National Sleep Foundation recommends avoiding chocolate before bedtime.[549] Not only is chocolate high in sugar (which affects the dopamine, serotonin, and melatonin levels in your brain), it also contains caffeine. Caffeine increases your cortisol levels to stay awake and alert, and we know that cortisol is inversely related to melatonin. Caffeine suppresses the production of melatonin, resulting in troubled sleep.

The tradition of eating dessert and watching television right before bed is a recipe for disaster. We already noted that inflammation associated with sugar intake is also responsible for the production of higher levels of cortisol, the hormone that contributes to stress and alertness. Stress is one of the most common reasons for troubled sleep. As the Mayo Clinic states, "Stressful times and events can cause temporary insomnia. And major or long-lasting stress can lead to chronic insomnia."[550] By adding in nighttime exposure to technology (e.g., television and cellphones), we are consistently interrupting our circadian rhythm through artificial

548 "Magnesium Rich Food," *Cleveland Clinic*, last modified November 24, 2020.

549 National Sleep Foundation, "How Much Caffeine Should You Really Be Having?," *Sleep.org*, accessed February 15, 2021.

550 Mayo Clinic Staff, "Insomnia," *Mayo Clinic*, October 15, 2016.

lighting. Exposure to light can suppress the production of melatonin, which makes it difficult to fall asleep. It is important to note that not all light has the same effect. In fact, blue light (wavelength range of 400-490nm) is the strongest, which means that the blue light from technological devices could have a significant impact on your circadian rhythm, affecting your ability to fall asleep.[551] The recent creation of blue light glasses has the public questioning the effects of these receptors. While some individuals believe it is not necessary to wear glasses if your vision is normal, recent science is explaining the benefits of blue-light glasses. Studies have reported a better quality of sleep for those who wear glasses to filter out blue light.[552]

ACID REFLUX

Sleeping and eating are not compatible. The digestive system's job is to turn our food into usable nutrients and energy.

For the Scientific Reader:

After ghrelin stimulates you to eat, another hormone, gastrin, is secreted due to the presence of food. Gastrin causes your stomach to produce acid, which aids in digestion.

If you think about it, when you go to sleep shortly after eating, your stomach is full of acid and food. Your mind should

---

551 Ibid; Guanluca Tosini et al., "Effects of Blue Light on the Circadian System and Eye Physiology," *Molecular Vision*, no. 22 (January 2016): 61–72.

552 Christopher M. Barnes, "Will Blue Light Glasses Improve Your Sleep?," *Harvard Business Review*, October 14, 2020.

automatically think of acid reflux here. It is surprising how our bodies can withhold from reflux the majority of the time after we eat before going to bed. One of the main functions of the esophagus is the acid esophageal clearance, which is composed of volume and chemical clearance. Volume clearance involves swallowing and peristalsis, the involuntary muscle contractions used to aid in moving food along the intestines. Chemical clearance uses saliva to neutralize the acid of the esophageal pH. When you are laying down and asleep, salivation is decreased, and gravity no longer assists peristalsis in moving food and acid down the esophagus and into the stomach. This leads to prolonged esophageal acid exposure time. You are more likely to experience acid reflux after eating if you choose to sleep on your back. The best sleeping position for people who experience acid reflux is on your left side. Sleeping on your left side is very different than on your right! While your esophagus is centered in your body, the stomach is curved placing a larger percentage on the left side. Sleeping on your right side allows for a more direct path for acid reflux to occur due to gravity and the stomach's curvature.[553] Raising your bed or using wedge pillows may also provide acid reflux relief. By elevating the head and chest, gravity hinders the ability for acid to travel back up and out through the esophagus.

ARE THERE BETTER FOODS THAN OTHERS TO EAT BEFORE BED IF HUNGRY?

Although most doctors recommend avoiding eating two to three hours before bed, if you are going to indulge in dessert right before bed, there are better foods than others to

---

553 "Heartburn Keeping You Up at Night?," *GI Society: Canadian Society of Intestinal Research*, accessed February 15, 2021.

consume. Foods high in potassium and B vitamins (like almonds and bananas) help the nervous system to relax. A food that is high in B vitamins, specifically B6, is chickpeas. Vitamin B6 aids in producing melatonin and serotonin. Surprisingly, foods can contain melatonin levels that may contribute to a better night's sleep. Foods high in melatonin consist of cherries, berries, and rolled oats.[554]

The amino acid tryptophan is the precursor for serotonin and melatonin. Increased levels of tryptophan would increase both serotonin and melatonin. Tryptophan is an essential amino acid that must be obtained through the diet, since humans cannot produce it. Salmon, chicken, spinach, and nuts are excellent sources of tryptophan.[555]

While it is unlikely chicken and salmon are consumed for dessert, cherries, berries, bananas, and nuts are more reasonable. Even if you cannot resist the sugar, choosing a cherry pie over a chocolate cake may help. The melatonin from cherries may result in less dramatic effects from the decreased serotonin from sugar.

Most of the time it is better to consume liquids instead of solids before bed. However, this needs to be evaluated very carefully. For example, ice cream/milkshakes should not be thought of as liquids. Even if it seems like a liquid when you consume it, by the time milk products reach the stomach, they form insoluble curd, making it hard for digestive enzymes to break down this solid. Ice cream is not the smartest dessert to eat before bed. It is solid for most of the

---

554 Jennifer Hines, "Food for Sleep: The Best and Worst Foods for Getting Sleep," *Alaska Sleep Education Center*, June 24, 2019.

555 Claire Sissons, "How to Boost Serotonin and Improve Mood," *Medical News Today*, July 10, 2018.

digestion. High-fat foods take longer to digest, so they sit in the stomach for longer periods. This may increase the stomach emptying time of two-and-a-half to three hours. The safest liquid is water and any flavor of it is safe, too.

The main exception to the rule is alcohol. Drinking alcohol is one of the worst things you can do for healthy sleep. While alcohol may have sedative effects that can make you feel tired and relaxed, it has been linked to poor quality of sleep.[556] Drinking alcohol before bed also increases your chances of acid reflux because alcohol relaxes the lower esophageal sphincter, the muscle that prevents acid reflux between the stomach and the esophagus.

Dessert, although referring to a sweeter course at the end of any meal, is most typically thought of as the last meal before sleep/the sweet meal after dinner. If you do decide to eat dessert, take a look at the clock. Learn how to optimize your eating schedule to minimize unwanted health effects associated with eating too close to bedtime.

---

556 Abhinav Singh, "Alcohol and Sleep," *Sleep Foundation*, last modified September 4, 2020; Michael D. Stein and Peter D. Friedmann, "Disturbed Sleep and Its Relationship to Alcohol Use," *Substance Abuse 26*, no. 1 (March 2005): 1–13.

EPILOGUE

Every day we are faced with the decision of when and what to eat. We have so many choices. I hope this book has challenged you to think about what you are putting into your body. Finding a diet and eating window that aligns with your needs and goals is a very individualized process. Even my twin brother who shares 50 percent of my DNA has completely different trigger foods than me.

I hope this is only just the start of your journey with food. Please use this book as a tool and reference when going out to explore on your own. Discuss your diet in conversations with your doctor about your medical concerns. Read the nutrition labels at grocery stores. Listen to your body; if you have a gut feeling about something, your gut microbiome may be trying to communicate with you. Spread awareness of the food-can-heal mindset to your friends and family. Let's normalize the idea that food can be used as medicine to improve our physical and mental health.

APPENDIX

INTRODUCTION

Anderson, David and Rebecca Wilkin. "Why So Many Americans Are Allergic to Peanuts." *Business Insider*, October 7, 2020. https://www.businessinsider.com/america-high-rate-peanut-allergies-compared-countries-2018-10#:~:text=So%2C%20what%20do%20these%20countries,is%20a%20popular%20peanuty%20snack.

Castles, Tom. "Pediatric Peanut Allergy Incidence and Prevalence on the Rise." *HCP Live*, November 17, 2018. https://www.hcplive.com/view/pediatric-peanut-allergy-incidence-and-prevalence-on-the-rise#:~:text=Pediatric%20Peanut%20Allergy%20Incidence%20and%20Prevalence%20on%20the%20Rise,-NOVEMBER%2017%2C%202018&text=Approximately%201.25%20million%2C%20or%202.2,and%20Immunology%20in%20Seattle%2C%20Washington.

Du Toit, George, Graham Roberts, Peter H. Sayre, Henry T. Bahnson, Suzana Radulovic, Alexandra F. Santos, Helen A. Brough, Deborah Phippard, Monica Basting, Mary Feeney,

Victor Turcanu, Michelle L. Sever, Margarita Gomez Lorenzo, Marshall Plaut, and Gideon Lack. "Randomized Trial of Peanut Consumption in Infants at Risk for Peanut Allergy." *The New England Journal of Medicine 372*, no. 9 (February 2015): 803–813. https://doi.org/10.1056/NEJMoa1414850.

Hourihane, Jonathan O'brien, Rachel Aiken, Rita Briggs, Lesley A. Gudgeon, Kate E.c. Grimshaw, Audrey Dunngalvin, and Stephen R. Roberts. "The Impact of Government Advice to Pregnant Mothers Regarding Peanut Avoidance on the Prevalence of Peanut Allergy in United Kingdom Children at School Entry." *Journal of Allergy and Clinical Immunology* 119, no. 5 (May 2007): 1197–1202. https://doi.org/10.1016/j.jaci.2006.12.670.

Office of the Commissioner. "FDA Approves First Drug for Treatment of Peanut Allergy for Children." *U.S. Food and Drug Administration*, January 31, 2020. https://www.fda.gov/news-events/press-announcements/fda-approves-first-drug-treatment-peanut-allergy-children.

Prescott, Susan L., Ruby Pawankar, Katrina J. Allen, Dianne E. Campbell, John Kh Sinn, Alessandro Fiocchi, Motohiro Ebisawa, Hugh A Sampson, Kirsten Beyer, and Bee-Wah Lee. "A Global Survey of Changing Patterns of Food Allergy Burden in Children." *World Allergy Organization Journal* 6, (December 2013): 21. https://doi.org/10.1186/1939-4551-6-21.

Productions, Craig Miller. "Dr. Gideon Lack Discusses Prevention of Peanut Allergy." 2018, *Vimeo* video, 00:46, https://vimeo.com/220977999.

Sicherer, Scott H., Anne Muñoz-Furlong, James H. Godbold, and Hugh A. Sampson. "US Prevalence of Self-Reported Peanut, Tree Nut, and Sesame Allergy: 11-Year Follow-Up." *Journal of Allergy and Clinical Immunology* 125, no. 6 (June 2010): 1322–26. https://doi.org/10.1016/j.jaci.2010.03.029.

The National Peanut Board. "Managing Peanut Allergies: A Resource for Parents, Educators and Others Who Care for Children." *Peanut Allergy Facts*, January 2015. https://peanutallergyfacts.org/resources/about-leap/#:~:text=A%20group%20of%20researchers%20from,approximately%2070%20to%2080%20percent.

Toit, George Du, Yitzhak Katz, Peter Sasieni, David Mesher, Soheila J. Maleki, Helen R. Fisher, Adam T. Fox, Victor Turcanu, Tal Amir, Galia Zadik-Mnuhun, Adi Cohen, Irit Livne, and Gideon Lack. "Early Consumption of Peanuts in Infancy Is Associated with a Low Prevalence of Peanut Allergy." *Journal of Allergy and Clinical Immunology* 122, no. 5 (November 2008): 984–91. https://doi.org/10.1016/j.jaci.2008.08.039.

Underwood, Trip. "Pregnancy and Peanuts: The End of the Avoidance Theory." *Boston Children's Hospital*, December 24, 2013. https://thriving.childrenshospital.org/pregnancy-and-peanuts-the-end-of-the-avoidance-theory/0/.

THE RISE OF NUTRITION

Flores, Mauricio, Gustavo Glusman, Kristin Brogaard, Nathan D Price, and Leroy Hood. "P4 Medicine: How Systems Medicine Will Transform the Healthcare Sector and Society." *Per-*

sonalized Medicine 10, no. 6 (August 2013): 565–76. https://doi.
org/10.2217/pme.13.57.

"From Feeding the US Army to Going to the Moon to Making
Everyday Moments G-r-r-r-Eat!." *Kellogg*. Accessed February
17, 2021. http://www.kellogghistory.com/history.html.

Institute of Medicine. *Front-of-Package Nutrition Rating Systems
and Symbols: Phase I Report*. Washington DC: National Academies Press, 2010.

Lucock, Mark. "Is Folic Acid the Ultimate Functional Food Component for Disease Prevention?." *BMJ 328*, no. 7422 (2004):
211–4. https://doi.org/10.1136/bmj.328.7433.211.

MNT Editorial Team. "What was Medieval and Renaissance Medicine?." *Medical News Today*, November 2, 2018. https://www.
medicalnewstoday.com/articles/323533.

National Archives. "White House Conference on Food, Nutrition
and Health (White House Central Files: Staff Member and
Office Files)." *Richard Nixon Presidential Library and Museum*,
accessed February 17, 2021. https://www.nixonlibrary.gov/find-
ing-aids/white-house-conference-food-nutrition-and-health-
white-house-central-files-staff.

Pike, Alyssa, Kris Sollid, and Ali Webster. "The Nutrition Facts
Label: Its History, Purpose and Updates." *Food Insight*, March
9, 2020. https://foodinsight.org/the-nutrition-facts-label-its-
history-purpose-and-updates/.

Price, Catherine. "The Age of Scurvy." *Science History Institute*, August 14, 2017. https://www.sciencehistory.org/distillations/the-age-of-scurvy.

Skrovan, Sandy. "The Origins and Evolution of Nutrition Facts Labeling." *Food Dive*, October 16, 2017. https://www.fooddive.com/news/the-origins-and-evolution-of-nutrition-facts-labeling/507016/#:~:text=In%201973%2C%20the%20FDA%20published,the%20label%20or%20in%20advertisin.

Taylor, Christine Lewis, and Virginia L. Wilkening. "How the Nutrition Food Label Was Developed, Part 1: The Nutrition Facts Panel." *Journal of the American Dietetic Association* 108, no. 3 (March 2008): 437–42. https://doi.org/10.1016/j.jada.2007.12.010.

"The History of Nutrition." *Natural Healers (Blog).* Accessed February 17, 2021. https://www.naturalhealers.com/blog/nutrition-history/.

"The Human Genome Project." *NIH: National Human Genome Research Institute.* Accessed February 17, 2021. https://www.genome.gov/human-genome-project.

"The Knight With the Lion: What Kind of Medicine Did People Use in the Middle Ages?." *University of Aberdeen.* Accessed February 17, 2021. https://www.abdn.ac.uk/sll/disciplines/english/lion/medicine.shtml.

Waxman, Henry A. "H.R.3562 - 101st Congress (1989–1990): Nutrition Labeling and Education Act of 1990." *Congress.gov,*

November 8, 1990. https://www.congress.gov/bill/101st-con-gress/house-bill/3562.

GUT MICROBIOME

Berdoy, M, J. P. Webster, and D. W. Macdonald. "Fatal Attraction in Rats Infected with *Toxoplasma Gondii.*" *Royal Society 267*, no. 1452 (August 2000). https://doi.org/10.1098/rspb.2000.1182.

Blader, Ira I., and Jeroen P. Saeij. "Communication between Toxoplasma Gondii and Its Host: Impact on Parasite Growth, Development, Immune Evasion, and Virulence." *Apmis* 117, no. 5–6 (May 2009): 458–76. https://doi.org/10.1111/j.1600-0463.2009.02453.x.

Chopra, Deepak. "What is the Secret to a Healthy Gut Microbi-ome?." *Chopra*, June 7, 2018. https://chopra.com/articles/what-is-the-secret-to-a-healthy-gut-microbiome.

Ferguson, James M. "SSRI Antidepressant Medications: Adverse Effects and Tolerability." *Primary Care Companion to the Journal of Clinical Psychiatry 3*, no. 1 (2001): 22–27. https://doi.org/10.4088/pcc.v03n0105.

Fields, Helen. "The Gut: Where Bacteria and Immune System Meet." *John Hopkins Medicine*, November 2015. https://www.hopkinsmedicine.org/research/advancements-in-research/fundamentals/in-depth/the-gut-where-bacteria-and-immune-system-meet.

Gatkowska, Justyna, Marek Wieczorek, Bozena Dziadek, Katarzyna Dzitko, and Henryka Dlugonska. "Behavioral

Changes in Mice Caused by Toxoplasma Gondii Invasion of Brain." *Parasitology Research 111*, (July 2012): 53–58. https://doi.org/10.1007/s00436-011-2800-y.

Gershon, Michael D. "5-Hydroxytrptamine (Serotonin) in the Gastrointestinal Tract." *Current Opinion in Endocrinology, Diabetes, and Obesity 20*, no. 1 (July 2013): 14–21. https://doi.org/10.1097/MED.0b013e32835bc703.

Global Health, Division of Parasitic Diseases and Malaria. "CDC - Toxoplasmosis - General Information - Frequently Asked Questions (FAQs)." *Centers for Disease Control and Prevention*, last modified September 3, 2020. https://www.cdc.gov/parasites/toxoplasmosis/gen_info/faqs.html.

Houghteling, Pearl D., and W. Allan Walker. "Why Is Initial Bacterial Colonization of the Intestine Important to Infants' and Children's Health?." *Journal of Pediatric Gastroenterology and Nutrition 60*, no. 3 (March 2015): 294–307. https://doi.org/10.1097/mpg.0000000000000597.

Janssen, P., R. Vos, and J. Tack. "The Influence of Citalopram on Interdigestive Gastrointestinal Motility in Man." *Alimentary Pharmacology & Therapeutics 32*, no. 2 (2010): 289–295. https://doi.org/10.1111/j.1365-2036.2010.04351.x.

Nobel Lecture. "Ilya Mechnikov: Nobel Lecture." *The Nobel Prize*, December 11, 1908. https://www.nobelprize.org/prizes/medicine/1908/mechnikov/lecture/.

Racine, Valerie. "Ilya Ilyich Mechnikov (Elie Metchnikoff) (1845–1916)." *The Embryo Project Encyclopedia*, July 5, 2014. https://

embryo.asu.edu/pages/ilya-ilyich-mechnikov-elie-metch-nikoff-1845-1916.

Robertson, Ruairi. "The Gut-Brain Connection: How It Works and the Role of Nutrition." *Healthline,* last modified August 20, 2020. https://www.healthline.com/nutrition/gut-brain-connection#TOC_TITLE_HDR_2.

Santarsieri, Daniel, and Thomas L. Schwartz. "Antidepressant Efficacy and Side-Effect Burden: A Quick Guide for Clinicians." *Drugs in Context 4,* no. 212290 (October 2015) https://doi.org/10.7573/dic.212290.

Sender, Rob, Shai Fuchs, and Ron Milo. "Revised Estimates for the Number of Human and Bacteria Cells in the Body." *PLoS Biology 14,* no. 8 (August 2016): e1002533. https://doi.org/10.1371/journal.pbio.1002533.

Scrvick, Kelly, Meredith Wadman, Jeffrey Brainard, Erik Stokstad, Kai Kupferschmidt, Sofia Moutinho, Jon Cohen, Sofia Moutinho, Sofia Moutinho, Sofia Moutinho and Lucy Hicks. *Brain Parasite May Strip Away Rodents' Fear of Predators-Not Just of Cats.* Science Magazine, January 14, 2020. https://www.sciencemag.org/news/2020/01/brain-parasite-may-strip-away-rodents-fear-predators-not-just-cats.

Spizman, Jocelyn. "Allergies, Asthma, and C-sections: The Implications of Birthing Methods." *Exploring Health,* October 20, 2020. http://exploringhealth.org/2020/10/20/allergies-asthma-and-c-sections-the-implications-of-birthing-methods/.

Stoller-Conrad, Jessica. "Microbes Help Produce Serotonin in Gut." *California Institute of Technology*, April 9, 2015. https://www.caltech.edu/about/news/microbes-help-produce-serotonin-gut-46495.

TED. "Ruairi Robertson: Food for Thought: How Your Belly Controls Your Brain," December 7, 2015, video, 14:30. https://www.youtube.com/watch?v=awtmTJW9ic8.

Turnbaugh, Peter J., Micah Hamady, Tanya Yatsunenko, Brandi L. Cantarel, Alexis Duncan, Ruth E. Ley, Mitchell L. Sogin, William J. Jones, Bruce A. Roe, Jason P. Affourtit, Michael Egholm, Bernard Henrissat, Andrew C. Heath, Rob Knight, and Jeffrey I. Gordon. "A Core Gut Microbiome in Obese and Lean Twins." *Nature* 457, no. 7228 (November 30, 2008): 480–84. https://doi.org/10.1038/nature07540.

INFLAMMATION

"Abundant Protein." *International Journal of Applied Biology and Pharmaceutical Technology.* Accessed February 15, 2021. https://www.iomcworld.org/medical-journals/abundant-protein-50938.html.

"Added Sugar in the Diet." *Harvard Health.* Accessed February 15, 2021. https://www.hsph.harvard.edu/nutritionsource/carbohydrates/added-sugar-in-the-diet/.

"Added Sugars on the New Nutrition Facts Label." *FDA.* Last modified March 11, 2020. https://www.fda.gov/food/new-nutrition-facts-label/added-sugars-new-nutrition-facts-label.

"Added Sugars." American Heart Association. Last modified April 17, 2018. https://www.heart.org/en/healthy-living/healthy-eating/eat-smart/sugar/added-sugars.

Alberts, Bruce, Alexander Johnson, Julian Lewis, Martin Raff, Keith Roberts, and Peter Walter. *Molecular Biology of the Cell, Fourth Edition*. New York: Garland Science, 2002.

An, Heejung. "Comparison of AGEs Produced by Different Cooking Methods." *Nongshim R&D*, November 8, 2013. https://icdm2013.diabetes.or.kr/slide/EC2-1%20Hee%20Jung%20An.pdf.

Anthony, Kiara. "How to Increase Stomach Acid at Home." *Healthline*, March 7, 2019. https://www.healthline.com/health/how-to-increase-stomach-acid.

Bender-Sibbio, Julie. "Could Hypochlorydria Be at the Root of Your Digestive Problems?." *JBS Nutrition and Wellness* (blog), November 28, 2017. https://www.jbsnourishwell.com/hypochlorydria-root-digestive-problem/.

Bickel, M. "The role of interleukin-8 in inflammation and mechanisms of regulation." *Journal of Periodontology* vol. 64, no. 5 (May 1993): 456–60. https://pubmed.ncbi.nlm.nih.gov/8315568/.

Bray, George A., Samara Joy Nielsen, and Barry M. Popkin. "Consumption of High-Fructose Corn Syrup in Beverages May Play A Role in the Epidemic of Obesity." *The American Journal of Clinical Nutrition 79*, no. 4 (2004): 537-543. https://doi.org/10.1093/ajcn/79.4.537.

Bui, Chumjit, Jerrold Petrofsky, Lee Bark, David Shavlik, Wilton Remigio, and Susanna Montgomery. "Acute Effect of a Single High-fat Meal on Forearm Blood Flow, Blood Pressure and Heart Rate in Healthy Male Asians and Causasians: A Pilot Study." *Southeast Asian Journal of Tropical Medicine and Public Health 41*, no. 2 (March 2010): 490–500. https://www.ncbi.nlm.nih.gov/pmc/articles/PMC3170142/.

Canales, Sarah Basford. "How to Cut Back on Red Meat Without Feeling Hungry All the Time." *Lifehacker*, September 4, 2020. https://www.lifehacker.com.au/2020/09/how-to-cut-back-on-red-meat-without-feeling-hungry-all-the-time/.

Connor, James R., Paul J. Beisswenger, and Benjamin S. Szwergold. "Some Clues as to the Regulation, Expression, Function, and Distribution of Fructosamine-3-Kinase and Fructosamine-3-Kinase-Related Protein." *Ann N. Y. Acad Sci 1043*, (June 2005): 824–36. https://doi.org/10.1196/annals.1333.095.

Crescendo Interactive Inc. "Dr. William "Buddy" Marterre Jr. (MDIV'17, P'05) & Ms. Roxanne Marterre (MDIV'17, P'19)." *Wake Forest University: Wake Will Lead* Accessed January 17, 2021. http://wfugift.org/?pageID=3&storyNum=12.

Daley, Cynthia A, Amber Abbott, Patrick S Doyle, Glenn A Nader, and Stephanie Larson. "A Review of Fatty Acid Profiles and Antioxidant Content in Grass-Fed and Grain-Fed Beef." *Nutrition Journal 9*, no. 10 (March 2010). https://doi.org/10.1186/1475-2891-9-10.

Danby, F. William. "Nutrition and Aging Skin: Sugar and Glycation." *Clinics in Dermatology 28*, no. 4 (July-August 2010): 409-411. https://doi.org/10.1016/j.clindermatol.2010.03.018.

DeLauer, Thomas. "Carbs and Inflammation: How Sugar Causes Inflammation." August 1, 2017, video, 5:29. https://www.youtube.com/watch?v=bmFlh3TgC50&list=WL&index=12.

DeLauer, Thomas. "What Sugar Does to Your Brain & Body: The Truth About Sugar." January 22, 2018, video, 7:10. https://www.youtube.com/watch?v=hElUqtRW1BQ.

"Diabetes: Rates of New Diagnosed Cases of Type 1 and Types 2 Diabetes Continue to Rise Among Children, Teens." *Centers for Disease Control and Prevention*. Last modified February 11, 2020. https://www.cdc.gov/diabetes/research/reports/children-diabetes-rates-rise.html.

Faruque, Samir, Janice Tong, Vuk Lacmanovic, Christiana Agbonghae, Dulce M. Minaya, and Krzysztof Czaja. "The Dose Makes the Poison: Sugar and Obesity in the United States – A Review." *Polish Journal of Food and Nutrition Sciences 69*, no. 3 (2019): 219–233. https://doi.org/10.31883/pjfns/110735.

Fessel Gion, Yufei Li, Vincent Diederich, Manuel Guizar-Sicairos, Philipp Schneider, David R. Sell, Vincent M. Monnier, and Jess G. Snedeker. "Advanced Glycation End-Products Reduce Collagen Molecular Sliding to Affect Collagen Fibril Damage Mechanisms but Not Stiffness." *Plos One*, November 3, 2014. https://doi.org/10.1371/journal.pone.0110948.

"Fruit Enzymes Tenderise Meat." *Science Learning Hub.* Accessed February 24, 2021. https://www.sciencelearn.org.nz/resources/1945-fruit-enzymes-tenderise-meat.

Fung, Jacqueline. "Nutrient and Health - Carbohydrates: Sugars." *Food Safety Focus.* Last modified November 16, 2018. https://www.cfs.gov.hk/english/multimedia/multimedia_pub/multi-media_pub_fsf_31_02.html.

Gabay, Cem. "Interleukin-6 and Chronic Inflammation." *Arthritis Research & Therapy* 8, no. 2 (July 28, 2006). https://doi.org/10.1186/ar1917.

Gancevicience, Ruta, Aikaterini I. Liakou, Athanasios Theodoridis, Evgenia Makrantonaki, and Christos C. Zouboulis. "Skin Anti-Aging Strategies." *Dermato-Endocrinology 4*, no. 3 (July 2012): 308-19. https://doi.org/10.4161/derm.22804.

Gaskins, Audrey J., Sunni L. Mumford, Alisha J. Rovner, Cuilin Zhang, Liwei Chen, Jean Wactawski-Wende, Neil J. Perkins, Enrique F. Schisterman, and the BioCycle Study Group. "Whole Grains are Associated with Serum Concentrations of High Sensitivity C-Reactive Protein among Premenopausal Women." *The Journal of Nutrition 140*, no. 9 (September 2010): 1669–1676. https://doi.org/10.3945/jn.110.124164.

Goldfein, Kara R., and Joanne L. Slavin. "Why Sugar Is Added to Food: Food Science 101." *Comprehensive Reviews in Food Science and Food Safety* 14, no. 5 (August 3, 2015): 644–56. https://doi.org/10.1111/1541-4337.12151.

Hannou, Sarah A., Danielle E. Haslam, Nicola M. McKeown, and Mark A. Herman. "Fructose Metabolism and Metabolic Disease." *The Journal of Clinical Investigation* 128, no. 2 (February 2018): 545–555. https://doi.org/10.1172/JCI96702.

"Health Warning for High-Heat Meat." *Hospital And Healthcare*, September 8, 2020. https://www.hospitalhealth.com.au/content/aged-allied-health/news/health-warning-for-high-heat-meat-621527120#axzz6ZjjVcYnS.

Ibrahim, José Noel, Isabelle Jéru, Jean-Claude Lecron, and Myrna Medlej-Hashim. "Cytokine Signatures in Hereditary Fever Syndromes (HFS)." *Cytokine & Growth Factor Reviews* 33 (February 2017): 19–34. https://doi.org/10.1016/j.cytogfr.2016.11.001.

IOS Press BV. "New Study Postulates the Role of Dietary Advanced Glycation End Products in the Risk of Alzheimer's Disease." ScienceDaily, February 3, 2015. https://www.sciencedaily.com/releases/2015/02/150203094144.htm.

Jourdan, Michel, Régis Bataille, Jacques Seguin, Xue Guang Zhang, Paul André Chaptal, and Bernard Klein. "Constitutive Production of Interleukin-6 and Immunologic Features in Cardiac Myxomas." *Arthritis & Rheumatism* 33, no. 3 (March 1990): 398–402. https://doi.org/10.1002/art.1780330313.

Jungen, Maarten J., Bastiaan C. Ter Meulen, Tim Van Osch, Henry C. Weinstein, and Raymond W. J. G. Ostelo. "Inflammatory Biomarkers in Patieents with Sciatica: A Systematic Review." *BMS Musculoskeletal Disorders* 20, no. 1 (April 9, 2019):156. https://doi.org/10.1186/s12891-019-2541-0.

Kahn, Joel. "TMAO: What We We Eat and What's Eating Us." Dr. Joel Kahn, *Huffington Post*, July 11, 2016. https://www.drjoelkahn.com/tmao-eat-whats-eating-us/.

Kany, Shinwan, Jan Tilmann Vollrath, and Borna Relja. "Cytokines in Inflammatory Disease." *International Journal of Molecular Sciences* 20, no. 23 (November 28, 2019): 6008. https://doi.org/10.3390/ijms20236008.

Kapil, Vikas, Rayomand S. Khambata, Amy Robertson, Mark J. Caulfield, and Amrita Aahluwalia. "Dietary Nitrate Provides Sustained Blood Pressure Lowering in Hypertensive Patients." *American Heart Association: Hypertension 65*, no. 2 (February 2015): 320–7. https://doi.org/10.1161/HYPERTENSIONAHA.114.04675.

Kimmons, Rolaynne. "Sugar in Western Diets Increases Risk for Breast Cancer Tumor and Metastasis." *The University of Texas MD Anderson Cancer Center*, December 31, 2015. https://www.mdanderson.org/newsroom/sugar-in-western-diets.hoo-158992968.html.

Klein, Alice Victoria, and Hosen Kiat. "The Mechanisms Underlying Fructose-Induced Hypertension: A Review." *Journal of Hypertension 33*, no. 5 (February 2015): 912–920. https://doi.org/10.1097/HJH.0000000000000551.

Kramer, Nicole E., Victoria E. Cosgrove, Kiley Dunlap, Mehala Subramaniapilai, Roger S. McIntyre, Trisha Suppes. "A Clinical Model for Identifying an Inflammatory Phenotype in Mood Disorders." *J Psychiatric Research 113*, (February 2019):148–158. https://doi.org/10.1016/j.jpsychires.2019.02.005.

Landry, Alexander, Peter Docherty, Sylvie Ouellette, Louis Jacques Cartier. "Causes and Outcomes of Markedly Elevated C-Reactive Protein Levels." *Official Publication of The College of Family Physicians of Canada 63*, 3 (June 2017): e316–e323. https://www.ncbi.nlm.nih.gov/pmc/articles/PMC5471098/.

Lefevre, Michael, and Satya Jonnalagadda. "Effect of Whole Grains on Markers of Subclinical Inflammation." *Nutrition Reviews 70*, no. 7 (May 22, 2012): 387–96. https://doi.org/10.1111/j.1753-4887.2012.00487.x.

"Limit Red and Processed Meat." *World Cancer Research Fund International.* Accessed February 23, 2021. https://www.wcrf.org/dietandcancer/recommendations/limit-red-processed-meat.

Ley, Sylvia H., Qi Sun, Walter C. Willett, A. Heather Eliassen, Kanaa Wu, An Pan, Fran Grodstein, and Frank B Hu. "Associations Between Red Meat and Biomarkers of Inflammation and Glucose Metabolism in Women." *The American Journal of Clinical Nutrition 99*, no. 2 (February 2014): 352–360. https://doi.org/10.3945/ajcn.113.075663.

Loveridge, Joel. "Chemistry of Bees: Bee Stings." *School of Chemistry, University of Bristol.* Accessed January 17, 2021. http://www.chm.bris.ac.uk/webprojects2001/loveridge/index-page8.html.

Luan, Ying-yi, and Yong-ming Yao. "The Clinical Significance and Potential Role of C-Reactive Protein in Chronic Inflammatory and Neurodegenerative Disease." *Frontiers in Immunology*, no. 9 (June 2018): 1302. https://doi.org/10.3389/fimmu.2018.01302.

Lustig, Robert H., Laura A. Schmidt, and Claire D. Brindis. "Public Health: The Toxic Truth About Sugar." *Nature 482*, no. 7383 (2012): 27–29. https://doi.org/10.1038/482027a.

Marterre, Buddy. "Bee Stings: Immunology, Allergy, and Treatment." Accessed January 17, 2021. https://wncbees.org/wp-content/uploads/2014/08/Bee-Stings-Immunology-Allergy-and-Treatment-Marterre.pdf.

Mawer, Rudy. "6 Reasons Why High-Fructose Corn Syrup Is Bad for You." *Healthline*, September 27, 2019. https://www.healthline.com/nutrition/why-high-fructose-corn-syrup-is-bad#5.-Can-increase-the-risk-of-other-serious-diseases.

Mayo Clinic Staff. "C-Reactive Protein Test." *Mayo Clinic*, November 21, 2017. https://www.mayoclinic.org/tests-procedures/c-reactive-protein-test/about/pac-20385228.

Mayo Clinic Staff. "Cuts of Beef: A Guide to the Leanest Selections." *Mayo Clinic*, October 29, 2019. https://www.mayoclinic.org/healthy-lifestyle/nutrition-and-healthy-eating/in-depth/cuts-of-beef/art-20043833.

Monteiro, Rosário, and Isabel Azevedo. "Chronic Inflammation in Obesity and the Metabolic Syndrome." *Mediators of Inflammation 2010*, (July 2010): 289645. https://doi.org/10.1155/2010/289645.

Montonen, Jukka, Heiner Boeing, Andreas Fritsche, Erwin Schleicher, Hans-Georg Joost, Matthias B. Schulze, Annika Steffen, and Tobias Pischon. "Consumption of Red Meat and Whole-Grain Bread in Relation to Biomarkers of Obesity, Inflammation, Glucose Metabolism and Oxidative Stress." *European*

Journal of Nutrition 52, no. 1 (February 2013): 337–45. https://doi.org/10.1007/s00394-012-0340-6.

Moor, Ashley. "Bee Sting: This Is What Happens to Your Body When You Get Stung by a Bee." *BestLife*, May 2, 2019. https://bestlifeonline.com/bee-sting/?nab=1%29.

Nathan, Carl, and Aihao Ding. "Nonresolving Inflammation." *Cell Press 140*, no. 6 (March 2010): 871–882. https://doi.org/10.1016/j.cell.2010.02.029.

Nehring, Sara M., Amandeep Goyal, Pankaj Bansal, Bhupendra C. Patel "C Reactive Protein." StatPearls. *US National Library of Medicine*, June 5, 2020. https://www.ncbi.nlm.nih.gov/books/NBK441843/.

Patel, Kamal. "How Are Carbohydrates Converted into Fat Deposits?." *Examine*. Last modified February 1, 2013. https://examine.com/nutrition/how-are-carbohydrates-converted-into-fat-deposits/.

Patel, Kamal. "What is the Difference Between High Fructose Corn Syrup (HFCS) and Sugar?." *Examine*. Last modified January 13, 2020. https://examine.com/nutrition/difference-between-hfcs-and-sugar/.

Pinto, R. S., U. F. Machado, and M. Passarelli. "Advanced Glycation End Products as Biomarkers for Cardiovascular Disease: Browning Clarifying Atherogenesis." *Bionarkers in Medicine 14*, no. 8 (June 2020). https://doi.org/10.2217/bmm-2020-0060.

"Playing with the Fire of Inflammation." *Harvard Health*, October 10, 2019. https://www.health.harvard.edu/staying-healthy/playing-with-the-fire-of-inflammation

Pussa, Seppo. "Dietary Advanced Glycation End Products." *Acne Einstein*. Accessed February 15, 2021. https://www.acneeinstein.com/cfl/dietary-advanced-glycation-end-products/#gref.

"Red Meat, TMAO, and Your Heart." *Harvard Health*, September 2019. https://www.health.harvard.edu/staying-healthy/red-meat-tmao-and-your-heart.

Ritchie, Hannah, and Max Roser. "Meat and Dairy Production." *Our World in Data*. Last modified November 2019. https://ourworldindata.org/meat-production.

Rowan, Sheldon, Eloy Bejarano, and Allen Taylor. "Mechanistic Targeting of Advanced Glycation End-Products in Age-Related Diseases." *Bichimica et Biophysica Act (BBA) – Molecular Basis of Disease 1864*, no. 12 (December 2018): 3631–3643. https://doi.org/10.1016/j.bbadis.2018.08.036.

Ruiz-Núññz, Begoña, Janneke Dijck-Brouwer, and Frits A.J. Muskiet. "The Relation of Saturated Fatty Acids with Low-Grade Inflammation and Cardiovascular Disease." *The Journal of Nutritional Biochemistry 36*, (October 2016): 1–20. https://doi.org/10.1016/j.jnutbio.2015.12.007.

"Saturated Fat." *American Heart Association*. Accessed February 23, 2021. https://www.heart.org/en/healthy-living/healthy-eating/eat-smart/fats/saturated-fats.

Strober, Jordan W., and Matthew J. Brady. "Dietary Fructose Consumption and Triple-Negative Breast Cancer Incidence." *Frontiers in Endocrinology* 10 (June 12, 2019). https://doi.org/10.3389/fendo.2019.00367.

Sutter Health. "Chronic Inflammation: Impact of Inflammation on Your Body." August 30, 2012. Video, 4:02. https://www.youtube.com/watch?v=x3zpVT14PxQ&list=WL&index=11%29.

Ted-Ed. "Nicole Avena: How Sugar Affects the Brain." January 7, 2014. Video, 4:53. https://letstalkscience.ca/educational-resources/stem-in-context/how-sugar-affects-brain.

TEDx Talks. "Jody Stanislaw: Sugar is Not a Treat." December 12, 2017. Video, 15:31.https://www.youtube.com/watch?v=tic7X-3ET4gE.

"The Functions of Carbohydrates in the Body." *The European Food Information Council (EUFIC).* Last modified January 14, 2020. https://www.eufic.org/en/whats-in-food/article/the-basics-carbohydrates.

"The Silent Killer." *Trivita.* Accessed January 18, 2021. https://www.trivita.ca/silentkiller/.

The Source Chiropractor. "How Sugar Leads to Pain and Inflammation." October 7, 2016, video: 3:50. https://www.youtube.com/watch?v=VIww6j6jI6Q.

Turco, Serena Del, and Giuseppina Basta. "An Update on Advanced Glycation Endproducts and Athersclerosis." *BioFactors 38*, no. 4 (2012): 266–274. https://doi.org/10.1002/biof.1018.

U.S. Department of Health & Human Services. "Diabetes: Type 2 Diabetes." *Centers for Disease Control and Prevention (CDC).* Last modified May 30, 2019. https://www.cdc.gov/diabetes/basics/type2.html.

University of California Television. "Red Meat, Disease, and Inflammation." August 7, 2020. Video, 4:31. https://www.youtube.com/watch?v=8paHL_ok5vg.

Uribarri, Jaime, Weijing Cai, Melpomeni Peppa, Susan Goodman, Luigi Ferrucci, Gary Striker, and Helen Vlassara. "Circulating Glycotoxins and Dietary Advanced Glycation Endproducts: Two Links to Inflammatory Response, Oxidative Stress, and Aging." *J Gerontol A Biol Sci Med Sci* 62, 4 (April 2007): 427–33. https://doi.org/10.1093/gerona/62.4.427.

Uribarri, Jamie, Sandra Woodruff, Susan Goodman, Weijing Cai, Xue Chen, Renata Pyzik, Angie Yong, Gary E. Striker, and Helen Vlassara. "Advanced Glycation End Products in Foods and a Practical Guide to Their Reduction in the Diet." *Journal of the American Dietetic Association* 110, no. 6 (June 2010): 911–16.e12. https://doi.org/10.1016/j.jada.2010.03.018.

Vocabulary.com, s.v. "inflammation (n.)." Accessed January 17, 2021, https://www.vocabulary.com/dictionary/inflammation.

Wang, Zeneg, Elizabeth Klipfell, Brian J. Bennett, Robert Koeth, Bruce S. Levison, Brandon Dugar, Aariel E. Feldstein, Earl B. Britt, Xiaoming Fu, Yoon-Mi Chung, Yuping Wu, Phil Schauer, Jonathan D. Smith, Hooman Allayee, W. H. Wilson Tang, Joseph A. DiDonato, Aldons J. Lusis, and Stanley L. Hazen. "Gut Flora Metabolism of Phosphatidylcholine Promotes Cardiovascular Disease." *Nature* 472, no. 7341 (April 2011): 57–63. https://doi.org/10.1038/nature09922.

Well + Good. "A Dietitian's Guide to Eating for Inflammation: You Versus Food." November 29, 2019. Video, 5:48. https://www.youtube.com/watch?v=vojXdgL6nGs.

Whiteman, Honor. "Study Links High Sugar Intake to Increased Risk of Breast Cancer." *MedicalNewsToday*, January 4, 2016. https://www.medicalnewstoday.com/articles/304636.

Whitney E. RD. "The Truth About Meat + Inflammation." May 14, 2019. Video, 6:20. https://www.youtube.com/watch?v=B-pdFx_9w9E8.

Wu, Tianying, Samantha Sonoda, and Hongxia Liu. "Unprocessed Red Meat Intakes are Associated with increased Inflammation, Triglycerides and HDL Cholesterol in Past Smokers." *Nutrition & Dietetics 77*, no. 2 (June 2019): 182–188. https://doi.org/10.1111/1747-0080.12555.

Wu, Lingyun, Sugandha Saxena, Mohammad Awaji, and Rakesh K. Singh. "Tumor-Associated Neutrophils in Cancer: Going Pro." *Cancers 11*, no. 4 (2019): 564. https://doi.org/10.3390/cancers11040564.

Wu, Xinle, and Vincent M Monnier. "Enzymatic Deglycation of Proteins." *Arch Biochem Biophys 419*, no. 1 (November 2003): 16–24. https://doi.org/10.1016/j.abb.2003.08.011.

Yu, Xiao-Hua, Yu-Chang Fu, Da-Wei Zhang, Kai Yin, and Chao-Ke Tang. "Foam Cells in Atherosclerosis." *Clinica Chimica Acta*

424, (September 2013): 245-252. https://doi.org/ 10.1016/j. cca.2013.06.006.

GLUTEN AND GRAINS

"Avidin-Biotin Interaction." *ThermoFisher Scientific.* Accessed January 22, 2021. https://www.thermofisher.com/us/en/home/ life-science/protein-biology/protein-biology-learning-center/ protein-biology-resource-library/pierce-protein-methods/avi-din-biotin-interaction.html.

Bar-Sela, Gil, Miri Cohen, Eran Ben-Arye, Ron Epelbaum. "The Medical Use of Wheatgrass: Review of the Gap Between Basic and Clinical Applications." *Mini Reviews in Medicinal Chemistry 15*, no. 12 (2015): 1002–10. https://doi.org/10.2174/13895575 1512150731112836.

Barclay, Eliza. "Sensitive to Gluten? A Carb in Wheat May Be the Real Culprit." *NPR*, May 22, 2014. https://www.npr.org/ sections/thesalt/2014/05/22/314287321/sensitive-to-gluten-a-carb-in-wheat-may-be-the-real-culprit.

Beninicasa, Paolo, Beatrice Falcinelli, Stanley Lutts, Fabio Stagnari, and Angelica Galleni. "Sprouted Grains: A Comprehensive Review." *Nutrients 11*, no. 2 (February 2019): 421. https://doi. org/10.3390/nu11020421.

Berg, Eric. "Dr. Berg's Story." *DrBerg.* Accessed January 24, 2021. https://www.drberg.com/dr-eric-berg/story.

Berg, Eric. "Wheat- Health Destroyer or Body Healer?." December 31, 2012. Video, 8:28. https://www.youtube.com/watch?v=h-K111hngfoc.

Bhikaji, Pawar Kiran, Thakare Mangala P., Meshram Dnyaneshwar Sudhakar, Jadhao Manju Namdev. "The Effect of Wheatgrass Juice on Hemoglobin Level W.S.R to Samanya-Vishesha Siddhanta." *International Journal of Ayurveda and Pharma Research 3*, no. 7 (July 2015). https://ijapr.in/index,php/ijapr/article/view/11.

Biesiekierski, Jessica R., Evan D. Newnham, Peter M. Irving, Jacqueline S. Barrett, Melissa Haines, James D. Doecke, Susan J. Shepherd, Jane G. Muir, and Peter R. Gibson. "Gluten Causes Gastrointestinal Symptoms in Subjects Without Celiac Disease: A Double-Blind Randomized Placebo-Controlled Trial." *The American Journal of Gastroenterology 106*, no. 3 (March 2011): 508–14. https://doi.org/o.1038/ajg.2010.487.

Biesiekierski, Jessica R., Simone L. Peters, Evan D. Newnham, Ourania Rosella, Jane G. Muir, and Peter R. Gibson. "No Effects of Gluten in Patients with Self-Reported Non-Celiac Gluten Sensitivity After Dietary Reduction of Fermentable, Poorly Absorbed, Short-Chain Carbohydrates." *Gastroenterology 145*, no. 2 (May 2013): 320–8.e1-3. https://doi.org/10.1053/j.gastro.2013.04.051.

Böhles, H. "Antioxidative Vitamins in Prematurely and Maturely Born Infants." *International Journal for Vitamin and Nutrition Research 67*, no. 5 (1997): 321–8. https://pubmed.ncbi.nlm.nih.gov/9350473/.

Butler, Natalie. "Can You Actually Ingest Too Much Fiber?." *Healthline*, April 16, 2019. https://www.healthline.com/health/food-nutrition/too-much-fiber.

Byrd-Bredbenner, Carol, Gaile Moe, Donna Beshgetoor, Jacqueline Berning. *Wadlwar's Perspectives in Nutrition Ninth Edition.* New York: McGraw-Hill Education, 2012.

Cannons, Clive, Stephen Duffull, Stewart Jessamine, Dilky Rasiah, and Michael Tatley. "What is Bioavailability and Bioequivalence?." *Best Practice (Journal)* (July, 2009): 4–8. https://pharmac.govt.nz/assets/bpjse-generics-2009.pdf.

Choung, Rok Seon, Aynur Unalp-Arida, Constance E. Ruhl, Tricia L. Bratner, James E. Everhart, Joseph A. Murray. "Less Hidden Celiac Disease but Increased Gluten Avoidance Without A Diagnosis in the USA: Findings from the National Health and Nutrition Examination Surveys from 2009 to 2014." *Mayo Clinic Proceedings*, (December 2016): 30634–6. https://doi.org/10.1016/j.mayocp.2016.10.012.

"Clean" *Clean Program*. Accessed January 18, 2021. https://www.cleanprogram.com/pages/our-mission.

Cox, Peter. *You Don't Need Meat.* New York, NY: Thomas Dunne Books, 2002.

Cronkleton, Emily. "Wheatgrass Benefits: 11 Reasons to Enjoy." *Healthline*. Last modified on October 12, 2017. https://www.healthline.com/health/food-nutrition/wheatgrass-benefits.

D'Souza, Hector. "Vitamin B2." *NDHealth* Facts. Last modified March 17, 2014. http://www.ndhealthfacts.org/wiki/Vitamin_B2.

Doheny, Kathleen. "What's Behind the Gluten-Free Trend?." *WebMD Health News*, September 16, 2016. https://totalbody-herbs.com/index.php/author/healthnews/page/302/.

"Dr. Alejandro Junger." Goop. Accessed on January 18, 2021, https://goop.com/goop-authors/dr-alejandro-junger/.

"Fiber: Why It Matters More Than You Think." *Experience L!fe*. Accessed January 18, 2021. https://experiencelife.com/article/fiber-why-it-matters-more-than-you-think/.

Gearry, Richard B., Peter M. Irving, Jacqueline S. Barrett, Debbie M. Nathan, Sue J. Shepheerd, and Peter R. Gibson. "Reduction of Dietary Poorly Absorbed Short-Chain Carbohydrates (Fodmaps) Improves Abdominal Symptoms in Patients with Inflammatory Bowel Disease-a Pilot Study." *Journal of Crohn's & Colitis* 3, no. 1 (February 2009): 8–14. https://doi.org/10.1016/j.crohns.2008.09.004.

Gibson, Peter R., and Susan J. Shepherd. "Evidence-Based Dietary Management of Functional Gastrointestinal Symptoms: The FODMAP Approach." *Journal of Gastroenterology and Hepatology* 25, no. 2 (January, 2010). https://doi.org/10.1111/j.1440-1746.2009.06149.x.

"Global Gluten Free Products (Food) Market Size Will Reach USD 36 Billion by 2026: Facts & Factors." *GlobeNewswire*. Accessed February 15, 2021. https://www.globenewswire.com/

news-release/2020/11/09/2122635/0/en/Global-Gluten-Free-Products-Food-Market-Size-Will-Reach-USD-36-Billion-by-2026-Facts-Factors.html.

"Gluten-Free Products Market Size, Share & Trends Analyst Report By Product (Bakery Products, Dairy/Dairy Alternatives), By Distribution Channel (Grocery Stores, Mass Merchandiser), By Region, And Segment Forecasts, 2020-2027." *Grand View Research*, February 2020. https://www.grandviewresearch.com/industry-analysis/gluten-free-products-market.

"'Gluten-Free' Means What It Says." *FDA*. Last modified January 11, 2021. https://www.fda.gov/consumers/consumer-updates/gluten-free-means-what-it-says.

"Glycemic Index for 60+ Foods." *Harvard Health*. Last modified January 6, 2020. https://www.health.harvard.edu/diseases-and-conditions/glycemic-index-and-glycemic-load-for-100-foods.

"Grains." *Let's Eat Healthy*. Accessed January 22, 2021. https://www.healthyeating.org/nutrition-topics/general/food-groups/grains.

Green, Peter H. R., and Rory Jones. *Gluten Exposed: The Science Behind the Hype and How to Navigate to a Healthy, Symptom-Free Life*. New York: William Morrow and Company, 2016.

Grundy, Myriam M.-L, Cathrina H. Edwards, Alan R. Mackie, Michael J. Gidley, Peter J. Butterworth, and Peter R. Ellis. "Re-evaluation of the Mechanisms of Dietary Fibre and Implications for Macronutrient Bioaccessibility, Digestion and Postprandial Metabolism." *The British Journal of Nutri-*

tion 116, no. 5 (July 7, 2016): 816–833. https://doi.org/10.1017/
S0007114516002610.

Gunnars, Kris. "FODMAP 101: A Detailed Beginner's Guide."
Healthline, November 9, 2018. https://www.healthline.com/
nutrition/fodmaps-101.

Gunnars, Kris. "Why Ezekiel Bread Is the Healthiest Bread You
Can Eat." *Healthline*, May 22, 2018. https://www.healthline.
com/nutrition/ezekiel-bread.

Guthrie, Catherine. "The Truth About Refined Grains." *Experience
L!fe*, July 1, 2019. https://experiencelife.com/article/the-truth-
about-refined-grains/.

Halmos, Emma P., Victoria A. Power, Susan J. Shepherd, Peter
R. Gibson, Jane G. Muir. "A Diet Low in Fodmaps Reduces
Symptoms of Irritable Bowel Syndrome." *Gastroenterology
146*, no. 1 (January 2014): 67–75.e5. https://doi.org/10.1053/j.
gastro.2013.09.046.

"Health Foods." *Mayo Clinic*, April 5, 2019. https://www.mayoclinic.
org/healthy-lifestyle/nutrition-and-healthy-eating/multime-
dia/health-foods/sls-20076653?s=10.

"Heart Healthy Eating to Help Lower Cholesterol Level." *Cleveland
Clinic*. Last modified February 16, 2018. https://my.cleveland-
clinic.org/health/articles/17281-heart-healthy-eating-to-help-
lower-cholesterol-levels.

Helen West. "Does Fiber Relieve or Cause Constipation? A Critical Look." *Healthline*. Last modified September 15, 2016. https://www.healthline.com/nutrition/fiber-and-constipation-truth.

Hoang, V. T. Ho, John L. Sievenpiper, Andreea Zurbau, Sonia Blanco Mejia, Elena Jovanovski, Fei A Au-Yeung, Alexandra L. Jenkins, and Vladimir Vuksan. "The Effect of Oat β-Glucan on LDL-Cholesterol, Non-HDL-Cholesterol and ApoB for CVD Risk Reduction: A Systematic Review and Meta-Analysis of Randomised-Controlled Trials." *British Journal of Nutrition* *116*, no. 8 (October 11, 2016): 1369–1382. https://doi.org/10.1017/S000711451600341X.

Horlock, Claire. "Enzyme-Linked Immunosorbent Assay (ELISA)." *British Society for Immunology, Imperial College London*. Accessed January 22, 2021. https://www.immunology.org/public-information/bitesized-immunology/experimental-techniques/enzyme-linked-immunosorbent-assay.

"How Much (Dietary) Fiber Should I Eat?." *USDA*, July 17, 2019. https://ask.usda.gov/s/article/How-much-dietary-fiber-should-I-eat.

"How Much Fiber Do Children Need?." *Cleveland Clinic*, December 30, 2020. https://health.clevelandclinic.org/figuring-dietary-fiber-child-need/.

"How Proper Fiber Intake Can Change Your Life and Improve Your Diet." *NuGo Fiber*, November 1, 2016. https://www.nugofiber.com/blog/change-your-life-with-fiber/.

"How Soluble Fiber Lowers Blood Cholesterol." *Verywell Health*, November 13, 2019. https://www.verywellhealth.com/insoluble-or-soluble-fiber-which-lowers-cholesterol-697724.

Institute of Medicine. *Dietary Reference Intakes Proposed Definition of Dietary Fiber.* Washington DC: National Academies Press, 2001.

"Is Wheatgrass Gluten-Free?." *Beyond Celiac.* Accessed January 24, 2021. https://www.beyondceliac.org/gluten-free-diet/is-it-gluten-free/wheatgrass/.

Ivanoff, George. *Fiber (What's in My Food?).* Mankato, MN: Smart Apple Media, 2012.

Jampolis, Dr. Melina. "What Exactly Does Fiber Do." *CNN*, November 8, 2012. https://www.cnn.com/2012/11/08/health/jampolis-explains-fiber/index.html?hpt=hp_bn12.

"Key Findings: Folic Acid Fortification Continues to Prevent Neural Tube Defect." *Centers for Disease Control and Prevention (CDC).* Last modified November 3, 2017. https://www.cdc.gov/ncbddd/folicacid/features/folicacid-prevents-ntds.html.

Kuroishi, Toshinobu, Luisa Rios-Avila, Valeria Pestinger, Subhashinee S K Wijeratne, Janos Zempleni. "Biotinylation Is a Natural, Albeit Rare, Modification of Human Histones." *Molecular Genetics and Metabolism 104*, no. 4 (December 2011): 537–45. https://doi.org/10.1016/j.ymgme.2011.08.030.

Laitinen, O. H., V. P. Hytönen, H. R. Nordlund, and M. S. Kulomaa. "Genetically Engineered Avidins and Streptavidins." *Cellular* and *Molecular Life Sciences* 63, no. 24 (December 2006): 2992–3017. https://doi.org/10.1007/s00018-006-6288-z.

Larsen, Laura, ed. *Diet and Nutrition Sourcebook*. Detroit, MI: Omnigraphics Inc., 2011.

Lattimer, James M., and Mark D. Haub. "Effects of Dietary Fiber and Its Components on Metabolic Health." *Nutrients* 2, no. 12 (December 15, 2010): 1266–1289. https://doi.org/10.3390/nu2121266.

Liao, Xiaofeng, Melissa Makris, and Xin M. Luo. "Fluorescence-Activated Cell Sorting for Purification of Plasmacytoid Dendritic Cells from the Mouse Bone Marrow." *Journal of Visualized Experiments* 117, (November 2016): 54641. https://doi.org/10.3791/54641.

Lindshield, Brian. "1.3: Polysaccharides - Fiber." Medicine *LibreTexts*, August 14, 2020. https://med.libretexts.org/Under_Construction/Purgatory/Book%3A_Intermediate_Nutrition_(Lindshield)/02%3A_Macronutrient_Structures/2.01%3A_Carbohydrates/2.1E%3A_Polysaccharides/1.03%3A_Polysaccharides_-_Fiber.

Lobo, V., A. Patil, A. Phatak, and N. Chandra. "Free Radical, Antioxidants and Functional Foods: Impact on Human Health." *Pharmacognosy Reviews* 4, no. 8 (Jul-Dec 2010): 118–26. https://doi.org/10.4103/0973-7847.70902.

Ma, Yunsheng, Jennifer A. Griffith, Lisa Chasan-Taber, Barbara C. Olendzki, Elizabeth Jackson, Edward J. Stanek III, Wenjun Li, Sherry L. Pagoto, Andrea R. Hafner, and Ira S. Ockene. "Association Between Dietary Fiber and Serum C-Reactive Protein." *American Journal of Clinical Nutrition 83*, no. 4 (April 2006): 760-766. https://doi.org/10.1093/ajcn/83.4.760.

Mancino, Lisa, and Jean C. Buzby. "Americans' Whole-Grain Consumption Below Guidelines." *Economic Research Service: United States Department of Agriculture*, April 1, 2005. https://www.ers.usda.gov/amber-waves/2005/april/americans-whole-grain-consumption-below-guidelines/.

Mayo Clinic Staff. "Chart of High-Fiber Foods." *Mayo Clinic*, January 5, 2021.https://www.mayoclinic.org/healthy-lifestyle/nutrition-and-healthy-eating/in-depth/high-fiber-foods/art-20050948.

Mayo Clinic Staff. "Gluten-Free Diet." *Mayo Clinic*, December 19, 2019. https://www.mayoclinic.org/healthy-lifestyle/nutrition-and-healthy-eating/in-depth/gluten-free-diet/art-20048530.

Mayo Clinic Staff. "Metabolic Syndrome." *Mayo Clinic*, March 14, 2019. https://www.mayoclinic.org/diseases-conditions/metabolic-syndrome/symptoms-causes/syc-20351916.

Mayo Clinic. "Mayo Clinic Minute: The Truth About Gluten." December 14, 2015, video, 1:07. https://www.youtube.com/watch?v=T9VFaFN-lo4.

Merriam-Webster, s.v. "Superfood (n.)." Accessed February 19, 2021. https://www.merriam-webster.com/dictionary/superfood.

Mitchell, Stephanie, Allison Gomes, Rena Zelig, and Anna Parker. "Not All Grains Are Created Equal: Gluten-Free Products Not

Included in Mandatory Folate Fortification." *Current Developments in Nutrition 3*, no. 5 (May 2019). https//doi.org/10.1093/cdn/nzz020.

Morris, Rebecca. "What Does Vitamin B5 Do?." *Healthline*. Last modified August 15, 2018. https://www.healthline.com/health/vitamin-watch-what-does-b5-do.

Muir, Jane G., Rosmary Rose, Ourania Rosella, Kelly Liels, Jacqueline S. Barrett, Susan J. Shepher, and Peter R. Gibson. "Measurement of Short-Chain Carbohydrates in Common Australian Vegetables and Fruits by High-Performance Liquid Chromatography (Hplc)." *Journal of Agricultural and Food Chemistry 57*, no. 2 (January 2009): 554–65. https://doi.org/10.1021/jf802700e.

National Institutes of Health, *The National Academies: Dietary Reference Intakes for Thiamin, Riboflavin, Niacin, Vitamin B6, Folate, Vitamin B12, Pantothenic Acid, Biotin and Choline*. Washington DC: National Academies Press, 1998.

"Nutrient Deficiencies." *Gluten.org*. Accessed January 21, 2021. https://gluten.org/2019/10/17/nutrient-deficiencies/.

Olsen, Natalie. "How Wheat Germ Benefits Your Health." *Healthline*, September 17, 2018. https://www.healthline.com/health/wheat-germ-benefits.

Olsen, Natalie. "Phytonutrients." *Healthline*, May 25, 2019. https://www.healthline.com/health/phytonutrients.

"Overview of Food Ingredients, Additives & Colors." *FDA*. Last modified February 6, 2018. https://www.fda.gov/food/food-ingredients-packaging/overview-food-ingredients-additives-colors.

Park, Yikyung, Amy F. Subar, Albert Hollenbeck, and A Arthur Schatzkin. "Dietary Fiber Intake and Mortality in the NIH-AARP Diet and Health Study." *Archives of Internal Medicine 171*, no. 12 (June 2011): 1061–8. https://doi.org/10.1001/archinternmed.2011.18.

Pordes, Piriya Mahendra. "Vitamin B5 (Panthothenic Acid): Benefits, Best Sources, Dosage, Deficiency." *Netdoctor*, March 6, 2020. https://www.netdoctor.co.uk/healthy-eating/a10925/vitamin-b5-pantothenic-acid/.

"Prevention and Treatment of High Cholesterol." *American Heart Association*. Accessed January 18, 2021. https://www.heart.org/en/health-topics/cholesterol/prevention-and-treatment-of-high-cholesterol-hyperlipidemia.

Quan, Zhou, Jiang Wu, Jie Tang, Jia-Ji Wang, Chu-Hong Lu, and Pei-Xi Wang. "Beneficial Effect of Higher Dietary Fiber Intake on Plasma HDL-C and TC/HDL-C Ratio among Chinese Rural-to-Urban Migrant Workers." *Int. J. Environ. Res. Public Health 12*, no. 5 (April 29, 2015): 4726–4738. https://doi.org/10.3390/ijerph120504726.

Rana, Satyavati, Jaspreet Kaur Kamboj, and Vandana Gandhi. "Living Life the Natural Way- Wheatgrass and Health." *Functional Foods in Health and Disease 11*, (November 2011): 444–456. https://www.functionalfoodscenter.net/files/47516971.pdf.

Rath, Linda. "Can Increasing Fiber Reduce Inflammation?." *Arthritis Foundation*. Accessed January 18, 2021. https://www.arthritis.org/health-wellness/healthy-living/nutrition/anti-inflammatory/increasing-fiber.

"Rethinking Fiber and Hydration Can Lead to Better Colon Health." *Harvard Health*, August 2013. https://www.health.harvard.edu/diseases-and-conditions/rethinking-fiber-and-hydration-can-lead-to-better-colon-health.

Sano, T., S. Vajda, and C. R. Cantor. "Genetic Engineering of Streptavidin, a Versatile Affinity Tag." *Journal of Chromatography 715*, no. 1 (1998): 85–91. https://doi.org/10.1016/s0378-4347(98)00316-8.

Saunders, Kerrie K. *The Vegan Diet As Chronic Disease Prevention.* New York, NY: Lantern Books, 2003.

Scazzina, F., M. DalliAsta, M. C. Casiraghi, S. Sieri, D. Del Rio, N. Pellegrini, and F. Brighenti. "Glycemic Index and Glycemic Load of Commercial Italian Foods." *Nutrition, Metabolism, and Cardiovascular Diseases (NMCD) 25*, no. 5 (February 2016): 419–29. https://doi.org/10.1016/j.numecd.2016.02.013.

Semeco, Arlene. "The 19 Best Prebiotic Foods You Should Eat." *Healthline*, June 8, 2016. https://www.healthline.com/nutrition/19-best-prebiotic-foods.

Shepherd, Susan J., Miranda Lomer, Peter R. Gibson. "Short-Chain Carbohydrates and Functional Gastrointestinal Disorders." *American Journal of Gastroenterology 108*, no. 5 (April 16, 2013): 707–717. https://doi.org/10.1038/ajg.2013.96.

Singh, Mahendra P., Sibhashinee S. K. Wijeratne, Janos Zempleni. "Biotinylation of Lysine 16 in Histone H4 Contributes Toward Nucleosome Condensation." *Archives of Biochemistry and Biophysics 529*, no. 2 (January, 2013): 105–11. https://doi.org/10.1016/j.abb.2012.11.005.

Slavin, Joanne. "Fiber and Prebiotics: Mechanisms and Health Benefits." *Nutrients 5*, no. 4 (April 2013): 1417-35. https://doi.org/10.3390/nu5041417.

Srinivasan, V. Srini. "Bioavailability of Nutrients: A Practical Approach to in Vitro Demonstration of the Availability of Nutrients in Multivitamin-Mineral Combination Products." *The Journal of Nutrition 131*, no. 4 (April 2001): 1349S–1350S. https://doi.org/10.1093/jn/131.4.1349S.

Staudacher, H. M., K. Whelan, P. M. Irving, and M. C. E. Lomer. "Comparison of Symptom Response Following Advice for a Diet Low in Fermentable Carbohydrates (Fodmaps) Versus Standard Dietary Advice in Patients with Irritable Bowel Syndrome." *Journal of Human Nutrition and Dietetics: The Official Journal of British Dietetic Association 24*, no. 5 (October 2011) 487–95. https://doi.org/10.1111/j.1365-277X.2011.01162.x.

Stayton, P. S., S. Freitag, L. A. Klumb, A. Chilkoti, V. Chu, J. E. Penzotti, R. To, D. Hyre, I. Le Trong, T. P. Lybrand, and R. E. Stenkamp. "Streptavidin-Biotin Binding Energetics." *Biomolecular Engineering 16*, no. 1-4 (December 1999): 39-44. https://doi.org/10.1016/s1050-3862(99)00042-x.

Stevens, Cara J. "Health Benefits of Biotin." *Healthline*, March 8, 2019. https://www.healthline.com/health/the-benefits-of-biotin.

"Soluble and Insoluble Fiber Food List." *North Ottawa Wellness Foundation*. Accessed February 19, 2021. https://www.northottawawellnessfoundation.org/wp-content/uploads/2017/11/NOWF-Fiber-Content-of-Foods.pdf.

"The Lowdown on Glycemic Index and Glycemic Load." *Harvard Health*. Last modified April 10, 2020. https://www.health.harvard.edu/diseases-and-conditions/the-lowdown-on-glycemic-index-and-glycemic-load.

"Together We Can Discover the Causes of Birth Defects." *National Birth Defects Prevention Study (NBDPS)*. Accessed January 22, 2021. http://www.nbdps.org/index.html.

Trumbo, Paula, Sandra Schlickre, Allison A. Yates, and Mary Poos. "Dietary Reference Intakes for Energy, Carbohydrate, Fiber, Fat, Fatty Acids, Cholesterol, Protein and Amino Acids." *Journal of the American Dietetic Association 102*, no. 11 (November 2002): 1621–1630. https://doi.org/10.1016/s0002-8223(02)90346-9.

"Understanding FODMAPS." *Canadian Digestive Health Foundation*. Accessed January 21, 2021. https://cdhf.ca/health-lifestyle/understanding-fodmaps/.

"Vitamin B." *Better Health*. Last modified May 2020. https://www.betterhealth.vic.gov.au/health/healthyliving/vitamin-b.

"Vitamin B5 (Panthothenic Acid)." *Mount Sinai*. Accessed January 22, 2021. https://www.mountsinai.org/health-library/supplement/vitamin-b5-pantothenic-acid.

Ware, Megan. "Everything You Need to Know About Gluten." *MedicalNewsToday*, July 17, 2018. https://www.medicalnewstoday.com/articles/308449.

"What Is Wheat Germ and Why Should I Be Eating It?." *Bob's Red Mill*, January 31, 2019. https://www.bobsredmill.com/blog/healthy-living/what-is-wheat-germ-and-why-should-i-be-eating-it/.

"What Is a Whole Grain." *Oldways Whole Grains Council*. Accessed January 22, 2021. https://wholegrainscouncil.org/what-whole-grain.

"What Makes Superfood So Super?." *UCDavis*. Accessed on January 24, 2021. https://www.ucdavis.edu/food/what-makes-superfood-so-super/.

Whitney, Ellie, Sharon Rady Rolfes. *Understanding Nutrition Eleventh Edition*. Belmont, California: Wadsworth Publishing Company, 2008.

Wisely, Rene. "This Gaseous Culprit Could Be Causing Your Stomach Pain and Constipation." *Michigan Health*, January 8, 2018. https://healthblog.uofmhealth.org/digestive-health/gaseous-culprit-could-be-causing-your-stomach-pain-and-constipation.

"What Are FODMAPS and What's the Connection to Celiac Disease and Gluten Sensitivity?." *Beyond Celiac*, October 28, 2015. https://www.beyondceliac.org/celiac-news/what-are-fodmaps-and-whats-the-connection-to-celiac-disease-and-gluten-sensitivity/.

"What Foods are in the Grains Group?." *MyPlate: U.S. Department of Agriculture*. Accessed on January 22, 2021. https://www.myplate.gov/eat-healthy/grains.

"Whole Grains A to Z." *Oldways Whole Grains Council*. Accessed January 22, 2021. https://wholegrainscouncil.org/whole-grains-101/whole-grains-z.

"Whole Grains, Refined Grains, and Dietary Fiber." *American Heart Association*. Accessed on January 18, 2021. https://www.heart.org/en/healthy-living/healthy-eating/eat-smart/nutrition-basics/whole-grains-refined-grains-and-dietary-fiber.

"Whole Gains vs. Regular Grains: What's the Difference?." *The Mayo Clinic Diet*. Accessed on January 22, 2021. http://diet.mayoclinic.org/diet/eat/whole-grains-vs-regular-grains.

Wrong, O. M., C. J. Edmonds, and V. S. Chadwick. "The Large Intestine: Its Role in Mammalian Nutrition and Homeostasis." *Quarterly Journal of Experimental Physiology 67*, no. 2 (April 1982): 217. https//doi.org/10.1113/expphysiol.1982.sp002643.

Yellin Juliana. "Everything You Need to Know About Grains." *Food Insight*, June 27, 2017. https://foodinsight.org/everything-you-need-to-know-about-grains/.

Zeratsky, Katherine. "How Can Bread Be Labeled as Both White and Whole Wheat? Is White Whole-Wheat Bread a Healthy Choice?." *Mayo Clinic*, January 18, 2020. https://www.mayoclinic.org/healthy-lifestyle/nutrition-and-healthy-eating/expert-answers/whole-wheat-bread/faq-20057999.

"2015-2020 Dietary Guidelines." *Health.gov*. Accessed January 22, 2021. https://health.gov/our-work/food-nutrition/previous-dietary-guidelines/2015.

FATS

Arnarson, Atli. "5 Studies on Saturated Fat- Time to Retire the Myth?." *Healthline*, February 20, 2020. https://www.healthline.com/nutrition/5-studies-on-saturated-fat.

"Ask the Doctor: Does "No Trans Fat" Really Mean No Trans Fat?." *Harvard Health*, October, 2006. https://www.health.harvard.cdu/newsletter_article/ask-the-doctor-does-no-trans-fat-really-mean-no-trans-fat.

Barnard, Neal. "Power Foods for the Brain." Tedx Talks, September 20, 2016. Video, 17:00. https://www.youtube.com/watch?v=v_ONFix_e4k.

Bienias J. L., L. A. Beckett, D. A. Bennett, R. S. Wilson, and D. A. Evans. "Design of the Chicago Health and Aging Project (CHAP)." *Journal of Alzheimer's Disease 5*, no. 5 (2003): 349–55. https://doi.org10.3233/jad-2003-5501.

Blondeau, Nicolas, Robert H. Lipsky, Mileed Bourourou, Mark W. Duncan, Philip B. Gorelick, and Ann M. Marini. "Alpha-Linolenic Acid: An Omega-3 Fatty Acid with Neuroprotective Properties—Ready for Use in the Stroke Clinic?." *Biomed Research International 2015*, (February 2015): 519830. https://doi.org/10.1155/2015/519830.

Braarud, Hanne Cecille, Maria Wik Markhus, Siv Skotheim, Kjell Morten Stormark, Livar Froyland, Ingvild Eide Graff, and Marian Kjellevold."Maternal DHA Status during Pregnancy Has a Positive Impact on Infant Problem Solving: A Norwegian Prospective Observation Study." *Nutrients 10*, no. 5 (April 2018): 529. https://doi.org/10.3390/nu10050529.

BrainMD (Blog) "Omega-3 and Omega-6: Know the Difference." December 21, 2016. Accessed February 25, 2021. https://brainmd.com/blog/know-fatty-acids-omega-3-omega-6/.

Brighman, Emily P., Han Woo, Meredith McCormack, Jessica Rice, Kristen Koehler, Tristan Vulcain, Tianshi Wu, Abigail Koch, Sangita Sharma, Gregory Diette, and Nadia N. Hansel. "Omega-3 and Omega-6 Intakes Modifies Asthma Severity and Response to Indoor Air Pollution in Children." *American Journal of Respiratory and Critical Care 199*, no. 12 (July 2019): 1478-1486. https://doi.org/10.1164/rccm.201808-1474OC.

Caporuscio, Jessica. "What Are the Most Healthful Oils?." *Medical News Today*, March 30, 2019. https://www.medicalnewstoday.com/articles/324844.

"Cell Membrane Fluidity." *Khan Academy*. Accessed February 15, 2021. https://www.khanacademy.org/test-prep/mcat/cells/cell-membrane-overview/v/cell-membrane-fluidity.

"Chia Seeds." *Harvard Health*. Accessed January 27, 2021. https://www.hsph.harvard.edu/nutritionsource/food-features/chia-seeds/.

Chrysohoou, Christina, Demosthenes B. Panagiotakos, Christos Pitsavos, Undurti N. Das, and Christodoulos Stefanadis. "Adherence to the Mediterranean Diet Attenuates Inflammation and Coagulation Process in Healthy Adults: The ATTICA Study." *Journal of the American College of Cardiology 44*, no. 1 (July 2004): 152–158. https://doi.org/10.1016/j.jacc.2004.03.039.

Cut. "Fat| Eating Disorders| One Word| Cut." February 22, 2016, video, 2:42. https://www.youtube.com/watch?v=UWX-wIPs-xWg.

De Alzaa F., Guillaume C., and Ravetti L. "Evaluation of Chemical and Physical Changes in Different Commercial Oils During Heating." *Acta Scientific Nutritional Health 2*, no. 6 (June 2018). https://actascientific.com/ASNH/pdf/ASNH-02-0083.pdf.

Dias, C. B., R. Garg, L. G. Wood, and M. L. Garg. "Saturated Fat Consumption May Not Be the Main Cause of Increased Blood Lipid Levels." *Medical Hypotheses 82*, no. 2 (February 2014): 187–195. https://doi.org/10.1016/j.mehy.2013.11.036.

"Dietary Fats." *American Heart Association*. Accessed January 27, 2021. https://www.heart.org/en/healthy-living/healthy-eating/eat-smart/fats/dietary-fats.

"DKA (Ketoacidosis) & Ketones." *American Diabetes Association*. Accessed January 27, 2021. https://www.diabetes.org/diabetes/complications/dka-ketoacidosis-ketones.

Esposito, Katherine, Raffaele Marfella, Miryam Ciotola, Carmen Di Palo, Francesco Giugliano, Giovanni Giugliano, Massimo D'Armiento, Francesco D'Andrea, and Dario Giugliano. "Effect of a Mediterranean-Style Diet on Endothelial Dysfunction and Markers of Vascular Inflammation in the Metabolic Syndrome: A Randomized Trial." *JAMA* 292, no. 12 (September 2004): 1440–1446. https://doi.org/10.1001/jama.292.12.1440.

"Facts and Figures." *Alzheimer's Association.* Accessed January 29, 2021. https://www.alz.org/alzheimers-dementia/facts-figures.

Fan, Shelly. "The Fat-Fueled Brain: Unnatural or Advantageous?." *Scientific American* (blog), October 1, 2013. https://blogs.scientificamerican.com/mind-guest-blog/the-fat-fueled-brain-unnatural-or-advantageous/.

"Final Determination Regarding Partially Hydrogenated Oils (Removing Trans Fats)." *FDA.* Last modified May 18, 2018. https://www.fda.gov/food/food-additives-petitions/final-determination-regarding-partially-hydrogenated-oils-removing-trans-fat.

Garg, A. "High-Monounsaturated-Fat Diets for Patients with Diabetes Mellitus: A Meta-Analysis." *The American Journal of Clinical Nutrition 67,* no. 3 (1998): 577S–582S. https://doi.org/10.1093/ajcn/67.3.577S.

Gavin, Mary L. "What's Cholesterol?." *Kids Health*, September 2018. https://kidshealth.org/en/kids/cholesterol.html.

"Grants Funded." *The National Institute for Psychobiology In Israel.* Accessed on March 2, 2021.

Handschuh, Dawn. "Arachidonic Acid." *Nutrition Facts.* Accessed January 29, 2021. https://nutritionfacts.org/topics/arachidonic-acid/.

Hankenson, K. D., B. A. Watkins, I. A. Schoenlein, K. G. Allen, and J. J. Turek. "Omega-3 Fatty Acids Enhance Ligament Fibroblast Collagen Formation in Association with Changes in Interleukin-6 Production." *Proceedings of the Society for Experimental Biology and Medicine* 233, no. 1 (January 2000): 88–95. https://doi.org/10.1064/j.1525-1573.2000.22312.x.

"HDL (Good), LDL (Bad) Cholesterol and Triglycerides." *American Heart Association.* Last modified November 6, 2020. https://www.heart.org/en/health-topics/cholesterol/hdl-good-ldl-bad-cholesterol-and-triglycerides.

Hooper, Lee, Nicole Martin, Asmaa Abdelhamid, and George Davey Smith. "Reduction in Saturated Fat Intake for Cardiovascular Disease." *The Cochrane Database of Systematic Reviews* 6, (June 2015): CD011737. https://doi.org/10.1002/14651858. CD011737.

Horrobin, D. F. "Fatty Acid Metabolism in Health and Disease: The Role of Delta-6-Desaturase." *The American Journal of Clinical Nutrition* 57, no. 5 (May 1993): 732S–736S. https://doi.org/10.1093/ajcn/57.5.732S.

J. de Souza, Russel, Andrew Mente, Adriana Maroleanu, Adrian I. Cozma, Vanessa Ha, Teruko Kishibe, Elizabeth Uleryk, Patrick Budylowski, Holger Schünemann, Joseph Beyene, and Sonia S. Anand. "Intake of Saturated and Trans Unsaturated Fatty Acids and Risk of All Cause Mortality, Cardiovascular Disease, and Type 2 Diabetes: Systematic Review and Meta-Analysis of Observational Studies." *BMJ 351*, (August 2015): h3978. https://doi.org10.1136/bmj.h3978.

Jacobs, Andrew. "Trans Fats Should be Eliminated Worldwide by 2023, W.H.O Says." *NyTimes*, May 14, 2018. https://www.nytimes.com/2018/05/14/health/trans-fats-who-ban.html.

King, Bailey. "Unsurprisingly, the Ketogenic Diet Was the Most-Googled Diet in 2018." *Philly Voice*, December 18, 2018. https://www.phillyvoice.com/ketogenic-diet-most-googled-diet-2018/.

"Lipids." *Khan Academy*. Accessed January 27, 2021. https://www.khanacademy.org/science/biology/macromolecules/lipids/a/lipids.

Lorgeril, M. de, P. Salen, J. L. Martin, I. Monjaud, J. Delaye, and N. Mamelle. "Mediterranean Diet, Traditional Risk Factors, and the Rate of Cardiovascular Complications After Myocardial Infarction: Final Report of the Lyon Diet Heart Study." *Circulation 99*, no. 6 (February 1999): 779–785. https://doi.org/10.1161/01.cir.99.6.799.

Martins, Julian G. "EPA but Not DHA Appears to Be Responsible for the Efficacy of Omega-3 Long Chain Polyunsaturated Fatty Acid Supplementation in Depression: Evidence from a Meta-Analysis of Randomized Controlled Trials." *Journal of the American College of Nutrition 28*, no. 5 (October 2009): 525-42. https://doi.org/10.1080/07315724.2009.10719785.

Mayo Clinic Staff."Trans Fat Is Double Trouble for Your Heart Health." *Mayo Clinic*, February 13, 2020. https://www.mayoclinic.org/diseases-conditions/high-blood-cholesterol/in-depth/trans-fat/art-20046114.

Mischoulon, David. "Omega-3 Fatty Acids for Mood Disorders." *Harvard Health*. Last modified October 27, 2020. https://www.health.harvard.edu/blog/omega-3-fatty-acids-for-mood-disorders-2018080314414.

Mori, Trevor A., Valerie Burke, Ian B. Puddey, Gerald F. Watts, David N. O'Neal, James D. Best, and Lawrence J. Beilin. "Purified Eicosapentaenoic and Docosahexaenoic Acids Have Differential Effects on Serum Lipids and Lipoproteins, LDL Particle Size, Glucose, and Insulin in Mildly Hyperlipidemic Men." *The American Journal of Clinical Nutrition 71*, no. 5 (May 2000): 1085–1094. https://doi.org/10.1093/ajcn/71.5.1085.

Moumtaz, Sarah, Benita C. Percival, Devki Parmar, Kerry L. Grootveld, Pim Jansson, and Martin Grootveld. "Toxic Aldehyde Generation in and Food Uptake from Culinary Oils during Frying Practices: Peroxidative Resistance of a Mono-unsaturate-Rich Algae Oil." *Scientific Reports 9*, no. 1 (March 2019): 4125. https://doi.org/10.1038/s41598-019-39767-1.

"Omega-3 ALA." *California Walnuts*. Accessed January 27, 2021. https://walnuts.org/nutrition/nutrition-info/alpha-linolenic-acid/.

"Omega-3 Fatty Acids." *National Institutes of Health*. Last modified October 1, 2020. https://ods.od.nih.gov/factsheets/Omega3FattyAcids-Consumer/.

"Omega-3 Fatty Acids." *National Institutes of Health*. Last modified October 1, 2020. https://ods.od.nih.gov/factsheets/Omega3Fat-tyAcids-HealthProfessional/.

Ophardt, Charles, and Antonio Rodriguez. "Hydrogenation of Unsaturated Fats and Trans Fats." *Chemistry LibreTexts*. Last modified August 10, 2020. https://chem.libretexts.org/ Bookshelves/Biological_Chemistry/Supplemental_Modules_ (Biological_Chemistry)/Lipids/Fatty_Acids/Hydrogenation_ of_Unsaturated_Fats_and_Trans_Fat.

Patel, Kamal. "Fish Oil." *Examine*. Last modified January 6, 2021. https://examine.com/supplements/fish-oil/research/.

Perlmutter, David. *Grain Brain: The Surprising Truth about Wheat, Carbs, and Sugar—Your Brain's Silent Killers*. New York: Little, Brown and Company, 2013.

Praagman, Jaike, Joline WJ Beulens, Marjan Alssema, Peter L. Zock, Anne J. Wanders, Ivonne Sluijs, and Yvonne T. Van Der Schouw. "The Association between Dietary Saturated Fatty Acids and Ischemic Heart Disease Depends on the Type and Source of Fatty Acid in the European Prospective Investigation into Cancer and Nutrition–Netherlands Cohort." *The American Journal of Clinical Nutrition 103*, no. 2 (February 2016): 356–365. https://doi.org/10.3945/ajcn.115.122671.

"Policies to Eliminate: Industrially-Produced Trans Fat Consumption." *World Health Organization*, 2018. https://www.who.int/docs/default-source/documents/replace-transfats/replace-act-information-sheet.pdf?ua=1.

Puori. "EPA and DHA Explained." June 29, 2018, video, 2:34. https://www.youtube.com/watch?v=LWoOAreKK7g.

Ramakrishnan, Usha, Ines Gonzalez-Casanova, Lourdes Schnaas, Ann DiGirolamo, Amado D. Quezada, Beth C. Pallo, Wei Hao, Lynnette M. Neufeld, Juan A. Rivera, Aryeh D. Stein, and Reynaldo Martorell. "Prenatal Supplementation with DHA Improves Attention at 5 Y of Age: A Randomized Controlled Trial." *The American Journal of Clinical Nutrition* 104, no. 4 (October 2016). 1075-1082. https://doi.org/10.3945/ajcn.114.101071.

Ramsden, Christopher E., Daisy Zamora, Boonseng Leelarthaepin, Sharon F. Majchrzak-Hong, Keturah R. Faurot, Chirayath M. Suchindran, Amit Ringel, John M. Davis, and Joseph R. Hibbeln. "Use of Dietary Linoleic Acid for Secondary Prevention of Coronary Heart Disease and Death: Evaluation of Recovered Data from the Sydney Diet Heart Study and Updated Meta-Analysis." *BMJ 346*, (February 2013): e8707. https://doi.org/10.1136/bmj.e8707.

Ramsden, Christopher E., Daisy Zamora, Sharon Majchrzak-Hong, Keturah R. Faurot, Steven K. Broste, Robert P. Frantz, John M. Davis, Amit Ringel, Chirayath M. Suchindran, and Josheph R. Hibbeln. "Re-Evaluation of the Traditional Diet-Heart Hypothesis: Analysis of Recovered Data from Minnesota Coronary Experiment (1968–73)." *BMJ 353*, (April 2016): i246. https://doi.org/10.1136/bmj.i246.

Sato, M., Y. Adan, K. Shibata, Y. Shoji, H. Sato, K. Imaizumi. "Cloning of Rat Delta 6-Desaturase and Its Regulation by Dietary Eicosapentaenoic or Docosahexaenoic Acid." *World*

Review of Nutrition and Dietetics 88, (2001): 196–9. https://doi.org/10.1159/000059780.

"Saturated Fat." *Heart UK*. Accessed January 29, 2021. https://www.heartuk.org.uk/low-cholesterol-foods/saturated-fat.

Sears, Barry. *Enter the Zone: A Dietary Road Map*. New York: Regan Books, 1995.

Sears, Barry. "What Are the Real Differences between EPA and DHA?." *Psychology Today*, April 1, 2012. https://www.psychologytoday.com/us/blog/in-the-zone/201204/what-are-the-real-differences-between-epa-and-dha.

Serhan, Charles N., Song Hong, Karsten Gronert, Sean P. Gronert, Pallavi R. Devchang, Gudrun Mirick, and Rose-Laure Moussigna. "Resolvins: A Family of Bioactive Products of Omega-3 Fatty Acid Transformation Circuits Initiated by Aspirin Treatment That Counter Proinflammation Signals." *The Journal of Experimental Medicine 196*, no. 8 (October 2002): 1025–37. https://doi.org/10.1084/jem.20020760.

Simopoulos, Artemis P. "The Importance of the Omega-6/Omega-3 Fatty Acid Ratio in Cardiovascular Disease and Other Chronic Diseases." *Experimental Biology and Medicine 233*, no. 6 (April 2008): 647-88. https://doi.org/10.3181/0711-MR-311.

Spencer, Elsa H., Hope R. Ferdowsian, and Neal D. Barnard. "Diet and Acne: A Review of the Evidence." *International Journal of Dermatology 48*, no. 4 (2009): 339–347. https://doi.org/10.1111/j.1365-4632.2009.04002.x.

Surette, Marc E. "The Science Behind Dietary Omega-3 Fatty Acids." *CMAJ: Canadian Medical Association Journal 178*, no. 2 (Jan 2008): 177–80. https://doi.org/10.1503/cmaj.071356.

"The Importance of Omega-3 and Omega-6 Fatty Acids." *Eufic*. Last modified March 27, 2019. https://www.eufic.org/en/whats-in-food/article/the-importance-of-omega-3-and-omega-6-fatty-acids.

Tutino, Valeria, Valentina De Nunzio, Maria Gabriella Caruso, Nicola Veronese, Dionigi Lorusso, Marta Di Masi, Maria Lucrezia Benedetto, and Maria Notarnicola. "Elevated AA/EPA Ratio Represents an Inflammatory Biomarker in Tumor Tissue of Metastatic Colorectal Cancer Patients." *International Journal of Molecular Sciences 20*, no. 8 (April 2019): 2050. https://doi.org/10.3390/ijms20082050.

Tutunchi, Helda, Alireza Ostadrahimi, and Maryam Saghafi-Asl. "The Effects of Diets Enriched in Monounsaturated Oleic Acid on the Management and Prevention of Obesity: A Systematic Review of Human Intervention Studies." *Advances in Nutrition 11*, no. 4 (July 2020): 864–877. https://doi.org/10.1093/advances/nmaa013.

University of Kansas. "DHA-Enriched Formula in Infancy Linked to Positive Cognitive Outcomes in Childhood." *ScienceDaily*, August 13, 2013. https://www.sciencedaily.com/releases/2013/08/130813101927.htm.

Van De Walle, Gavin. "Polyunsaturated Fats: Know the Facts About These Healthy Fats." *Healthline*, October 31, 2018. https://www.healthline.com/nutrition/polyunsaturated-fat.

Weatherby, Craig. "Omega-6 Overland Linked to Depression." *Vital Choice*, March 9, 2011. https://www.vitalchoice.com/article/omega-6-overload-linked-to-depression.

Weiser, Michael J, Christopher M. Butt, and M. Hasan Mohajeri. "Docosahexaenoic Acid and Cognition throughout the Lifespan." *Nutrients 8*, no. 2 (February 2016): 99. https://doi.org/10.3390/nu8020099.

Williams, C. M., J. A. Francis-Knapper, D. Webb, C. A. Brookes, A. Zampelas, J. A. Tredger, J. Wright, G. Meijer, P. C. Calder, P. Yaqoob, H. Roche, and M. J. Gibney. "Cholesterol Reduction Using Manufactured Foods High in Monounsaturated Fatty Acids: A Randomized Crossover Study." *The British Journal of Nutrition 81*, no. 6 (June 1999): 439–446. https://pubmed.ncbi.nlm.nih.gov/10615219/.

Winters, Diana R. H. "The FDA's Determination on Artificial Trans Fat: A Long Time Coming." *Health Affairs* (Blog), June 20, 2015. https://doi.org/10.1377/hblog20150623.048752.

Yang, Heng, Jiongxing Wu, Ren Guo, Yufen Peng, Wen Zheng, Ding Liu, and Zhi Song. "Glycolysis in Energy Metabolism During Seizures." *Neural Regeneration Research 8*, no. 14 (May 2013): 1316–1326. https://doi.org/10.3969/j.issn.1673-5374.2013.14.008.

Zeratsky, Katherine. "What Are MUFAs, and Should I Include Them in My Diet?." *Mayo Clinic*, April 28, 2020. https://www.mayoclinic.org/healthy-lifestyle/nutrition-and-healthy-eating/expert-answers/mufas/faq-20057775.

Zeratsky, Katherine. "What's an Easy Way to See How Much Fat I Eat Each Day?." *Mayo Clinic*, May 3, 2019. https://www.mayoclinic.org/healthy-lifestyle/nutrition-and-healthy-eating/expert-answers/fat-grams/faq-20058496.

"3 Ways DHA Supports Moms and Babies." *OmegaQuant*, February 12, 2019. https://omegaquant.com/3-ways-dha-supports-moms-and-babies/.

DAIRY

"A Guide to Foods Rich in Soy." *UCSF Health*. Accessed February 10, 2021. https://www.ucsfhealth.org/education/a-guide-to-foods-rich-in-soy/.

Abbott Laboratories. "Kefir Improves Lactose Digestion and Tolerance in Adults with Lactose Digestion." *Journal of the American Dietetic Association 103*, no. 5 (May 2003): 582-7. https://doi.org/10.1053/jada.2003.50111.

Adebamowo, Clement A., Donna Spiegelman, Catherine S. Berkey, F. William Danby, Helaine H. Rockett, Graham A. Colditz, Walter C. Willett, and Michelle D. Holmes. "Milk Consumption and Acne in Adolescent Girls." *Dermatology Online Journal 12*, no. 4 (May 2006): 1. https://pubmed.ncbi.nlm.nih.gov/17083856/.

Adebamowo, Clement A., Donna Spiegelman, Catherine S. Berkey, F. William Danby, Helaine H. Rockett, Graham A. Colditz, Walter C. Willett, and Michelle D. Holmes. "Milk Consumption and Acne in Teenaged Boys." *Journal of the American*

Academy of Dermatology 58, no. 5 (2008): 787–793. https://doi. org/10.1016/j.jaad.2007.08.049.

Adebamowo, Clement A., Donna Spiegelman, F. William Danby, A. Lindsay Frazier, Walter C. Willett, and Michelle D. Holmes. "High School Dietary Dairy Intake and Teenage Acne." *Journal of the American Academy of Dermatology 52*, no. 2 (February 2005): 207–214. https://doi.org/10.1016/j.jaad.2004.08.007.

Afeiche, M., P. L. Williams, J. Mendiola, A. J. Gaskins, N. Jorgensen, S. H. Swan, and J. E. Chavarro. "Dairy Food Intake in Relation to Semen Quality and Reproductive Hormone Levels among Physically Active Young Men." *Human Reproduction 28*, no. 8 (August 2013): 2265-2275. https://doi.org/10.1093/humrep/det133.

Bell, Becky. "Is Whole Milk Better Than Low-Fat and Skim Milk?." *Healthline*, October 26, 2016. https://www.healthline.com/nutrition/whole-vs-skim-milk.

"Bovine Somatotropin (bST)." *FDA*. Last modified April 21, 2020. https://www.fda.gov/animal-veterinary/product-safety-information/bovine-somatotropin-bst.

Breast Cancer Research Foundation. "If Most Breast Cancers Are Driven by Estrogen, Why Are Peak Incidences after Menopause?." April 10, 2014, video, 1:10. https://www.youtube.com/watch?v=foQ5b_HmWFk.

Brechon, Sarah. "Estrogen and Breast Cancer." *Maurer Foundation: Breast Health Education*, February 7, 2012. https://www.maurerfoundation.org/estrogen-and-breast-cancer/.

Cafasso, Jacquelyn. "10 Reasons to Take a Bifidus Probiotic."
Healthline. Last modified October 12, 2017. https://www.health-
line.com/health/food-nutrition/bifidus.

"Calcium and Bone Health." *Help Guide.* Last modified October
2020. https://www.helpguide.org/articles/healthy-eating/cal-
cium-and-bone-health.htm.

"Calcium and Your Child." *John Hopkins Medicine.* Accessed
February 3, 2021. https://www.hopkinsallchildrens.org/
Patients-Families/Health-Library/HealthDocNew/Calcium-
and-Your-Child.

"Calcium Content of Foods." *UCSF Health.* Accessed February
11, 2021. https://www.ucsfhealth.org/education/calcium-con-
tent-of-foods.

"Can People Who Are Lactose Intolerant Consume Milk Anyway?."
ProCon. Last modified April 9, 2008. https://milk.procon.org/
questions/can-people-who-are-lactose-intolerant-consume-
milk-anyway/.

Castro, Luiz Claudio, Alicia Diaz-Thomas, and Ramon Mar-
tinez. "Children and Bone Health." *Hormone Health Network.* Last modified July 2020. https://www.hormone.org/
your-health-and-hormones/children-and-teen-health/chil-
dren-and-bone-health#:~:text=The%20most%20important%20
time%20for,also%20get%20denser%20(thicker).

Cengiz, Fatma Pelin, Bengu Cevirgen Cernil, Nazan Emiroglu,
Anil Gulsel Bahali, and Nahide Onsun. "Acne Located on the
Trunk, Whey Protein Supplementation: Is There Any Associ-

ation?." *Health Promotion Perspectives 7*, no. 2 (March 2017): 106–108. https://doi.org/10.15171/hpp.2017.19.

Chen, George Q., Thomas S. H. Leong, Sandra E. Kentish, Muthupandian Ashokkumar, Gregory J. O. Martin. "Chapter 8 – Membrane Separations in the Dairy Industry." *Separation of Functional Molecules in Food by Membrane Technology* (2019): 267–304. https://doi.org/10.1016/B978-0-12-815056-6.00008-5.

"Coconut-Based Vanilla." *Chobani.* Accessed February 13, 2021. https://www.chobani.com/products/chobani-coconut/cup/vanilla/.

"Coconut Milk." *Califia Farms.* Accessed February 13, 2021. https://www.califiafarms.com/collections/plant-milks/products/go-coconuts-coconutmilk-48oz.

Cramer, Daniel W. Cramer, Huijuan Xu, and Timo Sahi. "Adult Hypolactasia, Milk Consumption, and Age-Specific Fertility." *American Journal of Epidemiology 139*, no. 3 (1994): 282–9. https://citeseerx.ist.psu.edu/viewdoc/download?-doi=10.1.1.917.771&rep=rep1&type=pdf.

Danby, William F. "Nutrition and Acne." *Clinics in Dermatology 28*, no. 6 (November-December 2010): 598-604. https://doi.org/10.1016/j.clindermatol.2010.03.017.

Davis, Carole, and Etta Saltos. "Dietary Recommendations and How They Have Changed Over Time." *Economic Research Service, U.S. Department of Agriculture*, 33–50. https://www.ers.usda.gov/webdocs/publications/42215/5831_aib750b_1_.pdf.

Fontecha, Javier, Maria Visitación Calvo, Manuela Juarez, Angel Gil, Vincente Martínez-Vizcaino. "Milk and Dairy Product Consumption and Cardiovascular Diseases: An Overview of Systematic Reviews and Meta-Analyses." *Advances in Nutrition* 10, no. 2 (May 2019): S164-S189. https://doi.org/10.1093/advances/nmy099.

"General Chemistry Lab Tutorials: Calcium in the Body." *Washington University St. Louis.* Accessed February 3, 2021. http://www.chemistry.wustl.edu/~edudev/LabTutorials/CourseTutorials/Tutorials/Vitamins/calcium.htm.

Glibowski, P., and A. Turczyn. "Determining the Effect of Consuming Fermented Milk Drinks on the Incidence of Constipation, Diarrhoea and Resistance to Respiratory Illness." *Roczniki Państwowego Zakładu Higieny* 64, no. 4 (2013). http://yadda.icm.edu.pl/yadda/element/bwmeta1.element.agro-222d65e4-dee5-42c8-942a-6ef2e86e9eac.

"Gut Feelings: The Power of Fermented Dairy." *The Guardian, Dairy Australia.* Accessed February 4, 2021. https://www.theguardian.com/dairy-australia-listen-to-your-gut/2019/jun/27/gut-feelings-the-power-of-fermented-dairy.

Haug, Anna, Arne T. Hostmark, and Odd M. Harstad. "Bovine Milk in Human Nutrition – A Review." *Lipids in Health and Disease* 6, no. 25 (September 2007). https://doi.org/10.1186/1476-511X-6-25.

"Health Concerns About Dairy." *Physicians Committee for Responsible Medicine.* Accessed February 11, 2021. https://www.pcrm.

org/good-nutrition/nutrition-information/health-concerns-about-dairy.

"Increasing Calcium in Your Diet." *Cleveland Clinic.* Last modified December 1, 2019. https://my.clevelandclinic.org/health/drugs/16297-increasing-calcium-in-your-diet.

"Katherine Isacks." *My Net Diary.* Accessed February 4, 2021. https://www.mynetdiary.com/bio-kisacks.html.

"Lactose Intolerance." *Medline Plus.* Last modified August 18, 2020. https://medlineplus.gov/genetics/condition/lactose-intolerance/#frequency.

Lanou, Amy Joy. "Should Dairy Be Recommended as Part of a Healthy Vegetarian Diet? Counterpoint." *The American Journal of Clinical Nutrition 89,* no. 5 (May 2009): 1638S–1642S. https://doi.org/10.3945/ajcn.2009.26736P.

Lim, Dr. Davin. "Skin Care Tips- Treating Hormonal Acne." May 20, 2018, video, 13:53. https://www.youtube.com/watch?v=zN-QdHr74R8Q.

Liu, G., G. E. Hale, and C. L. Hughes. "Galactose Metabolism and Ovarian Toxicity." *Reproductive Toxicology 14,* no. 5 (September-October 2000): 377-84. https://doi.org/10.1016/s0890-6238(00)00096-4.

"Live & Active Cultures Seal." *International Dairy Foods Association (IDFA).* Accessed February 4, 2021. https://www.idfa.org/live-active-cultures-seal.

Lordan, Ronan, Alexandros Tsoupras, Bhaskar Mitra, and Ioannis Zabetakis. "Dairy Fats and Cardiovascular Disease: Do We Really Need to Be Concerned?." *Foods 7*, no. 3 (May 2018): 29. https://doi.org/10.3390/foods7030029.

Makrantonaki, Evgenia, Ruta Ganceviciene, and Christos Zouboulis. "An Update on the Role of the Sebaceous Gland in the Pathogenesis of Acne." *Dermatoendocrinology 3*, no.1 (2011): 41–9. https://doi.org/10.4161/derm.3.1.13900.

Mayo Clinic Staff. "Lactose Intolerance." *Mayo Clinic*, April 7, 2020. https://www.mayoclinic.org/diseases-conditions/lactose-intolerance/symptoms-causes/syc-20374232.

Merriam-Webster, s.v. "Dairy (n.)." Accessed February 19, 2021. https://www.merriam-webster.com/dictionary/dairy.

"Milk for Your Bones?." *WebMD*, October 6, 2000. https://www.webmd.com/food-recipes/features/milk-for-your-bones#1.

"Oat Milk." *Califia Farms*. Accessed February 13, 2021. https://www.califiafarms.com/collections/plant-milks/products/oatmilk.

Palmer, Angela. "The Link Between Milk and Acne." *Verywell Health*. Last modified December 10, 2019. https://www.verywellhealth.com/does-drinking-milk-cause-acne-15684.

Physicians Committee. Neal Barnard, MD: How Food Affects Hormones. March 18, 2020, video, 54:19. https://www.youtube.com/watch?v=os5vzsabNpI.

Pointer, Kathleen. "Should You Remove Carrageenan from Your Diet?." *Healthline*. Last modified October 12, 2017. https://www.healthline.com/health/food-nutrition/carrageenan.

"Pregnant Cows, Timing of Pregnancy, Open Cows, Pregnancy Rate." *Institute of Agriculture and Natural Resources*. Accessed February 10, 2021. https://beef.unl.edu/faq/pregnant-cows.

Rosa, Damiana D., Manoela M. S. Dias, Lukasz M. Grzeskowiak, Sandra A. Reis, Lisiane L. Conceicao, and Maria de Carmo G. Peluzio. "Milk Kefir: Nutritional, Microbiological and Health Benefits." *Nutrition Research Reviews 30*, no. 1 (February 2017): 82–96. https://doi.org/10.1017/S0954422416000275.

Shu, Xiao Ou, Ying Zhend, Hui Cai, Kai Gu, Zhi Chen, Wei Zheng, and Wei Lu. "Soy Food Intake and Breast Cancer Survival." *JAMA 302*, no. 22 (December 2010): 2437–2443. https://doi.org/10.1001/jama.2009.1783.

Simon, James. "Androgen." *Healthy Women*. Accessed February 11, 2021. https://www.healthywomen.org/your-health/androgen/diagnosis.

"The Nutrition Source: Calcium." *Harvard Health*. Accessed February 10, 2021. https://www.hsph.harvard.edu/nutritionsource/calcium/.

Torborg, Liza. "Mayo Clinic Q and A: Dairy Milk, Soy Milk, Almond Milk – Which is the Healthiest Choice for you?." *Mayo Clinic: News Network*, April 9, 2019. https://newsnetwork.mayoclinic.org/discussion/mayo-clinic-q-and-a-dairy-milk-soy-milk-almond-milk-which-is-the-healthiest-choice-for-you/.

"Unsweetened Almond Milk." *Califia Farms*. Accessed February 13, 2021. https://www.califiafarms.com/collections/plant-milks/products/unsweetened-48oz.

Ware, Megan. "Everything You Need to Know about Yogurt." *Medical News Today*, January 11, 2018. https://www.medicalnewstoday.com/articles/295714.

"What is the Lactose Content of Different Dairy Products?." *Dairy Australia*. Last modified September 18, 2019. https://www.dairy.com.au/dairy-matters/you-ask-we-answer/what-is-the-lactose-content-of-different-dairy-products.

"Whole Milk Plain Greek Yogurt." *Chobani*. Accessed February 13, 2021. https://www.chobani.com/products/plain/large-size-tub/whole-milk-plain/.

"Yogurt." *Harvard Health*. Accessed February 4, 2021. https://www.hsph.harvard.edu/nutritionsource/food-features/yogurt/.

"Yogurt Production." *Milk Facts*. Accessed February 4, 2021. http://www.milkfacts.info/Milk%20Processing/Yogurt%20Production.htm.

SUPPLEMENTS

Alaimo, K., M. A. McDowell, R. R. Briefel, A. M. Bischof, C. R. Caughman, C. M. Loria, and C. L. Johnson. "Dietary Intake of Vitamins, Minerals, and Fiber of Persons Ages 2 Months and Over in the United States: Third National Health and Nutrition Examination Survey, Phase 1, 1988–91." *Advance*

Data 258, (November 1994): 1–28. https://pubmed.ncbi.nlm.nih.gov/10138938/.

Aloia, John F., Manish Patel, Rhett Dimaano, Melissa Li-Ng, Sonia A. Talwar, Mageda Mikhail, Simcha Pollack, and James K. Yeh. "Vitamin D Intakes to Attain a Desired Serum 25-Hydroxyvitamin D Concentration." *The American Journal of Clinical Nutrition 87*, no. 6 (June 2008): 1952-1958. https://doi.org/10.1093/ajcn/87.6.1952.

Anthony, Kiara. "High Homocysteine Level (Hyperhomocysteinemia)." *Healthline*. Last modified September 18, 2018. https://www.healthline.com/health/homocysteine-levels#symptoms.

"Antioxidants: In Depth." *NIH: National Center for Complementary and Integrative Health*. Last modified November 2013. https://www.nccih.nih.gov/health/antioxidants-in-depth.

Arterburn, Linda M., Harry A. Oken, Eileen Bailey Hall, Jacqueline Hamersley, Connye N. Kuratko, and James P. Hoffman. "Algal-Oil Capsules and Cooked Salmon: Nutritionally Equivalent Sources of Docosahexaenoic Acid." *Journal of the American Dietetic Association 108*, no. 7 (2008): 1204–1209. https://doi.org/10.1016/j.jada.2008.04.020.

Asher, Gary N., Amanda H. Corbett, and Roy L. Hawke. "Common Herbal Dietary Supplement-Drug Interactions." *American Family Physician 96*, no. 2 (July 2017): 101–107. https://www.aafp.org/afp/2017/0715/p101.html.

Bito, Tomohiro, Taihei Misaki, Yukinori Yabuta, Takahiro Ishikawa, Tsuyoshi Kawano, and Fumio Watanabe. "Vitamin

B12 Deficiency Results in Severe Oxidative Stress, Leading to Memory Retention Impairment in *Caenorhabditis Elegans.*" *Redox Biology 11*, (April 2017): 21-29. https://doi.org/10.1016/j.redox.2016.10.013.

Bodnar, Lisa M., Gong Tang, Roberta B. Ness, Gail Harger, and James M. Roberts. "Periconceptional Multivitamin Use Reduces the Risk of Preeclampsia." *American Journal of Epidemiology 164*, no. 5 (September 2006): 470–477. https://doi.org/10.1093/aje/kwj218.

Brocadello, Filippo, Giorgio Levedianos, Francesco Piccione, Renzo Manara, and Francesco Francini Pesenti. "Irreversible Subacute Sclerotic Combined Degeneration of the Spinal Cord in a Vegan Subject." *Nutrition 23*, no. 7–8 (July-August 2007): 622–624. https://doi.org/10.1016/j.nut.2007.05.006.

Brown, LaVerne L., Barbara Cohen, Derrick Tabor, Giovanna Zapplalà, Padma Maruvada, and Paul M Coates. "The Vitamin D Paradox in Black Americans: A Systems-Based Approach to Investigating Clinical Practice, Research, and Public Health - Expert Panel Meeting Report." *BMC Proceedings 12*, no. 6 (2018). https://doi.org/10.1186/s12919-018-0102-4.

Butler, Justine. "Essential Guide to Antioxidants on a Vegan Diet." *Plant Based News.* Last modified October 1, 2020. https://plantbasednews.org/lifestyle/essential-guide-antioxidants-vegan-diet/.

Campbell, J. K., and C. F. Mills. "Effects of Dietary Cadmium and Zinc on Rats Maintained on Diets Low in Copper." *The Pro-*

ceedings of the Nutrition Society 33, no. 1 (May 1974): 15A–16A. https://pubmed.ncbi.nlm.nih.gov/4418680/.

Cardwell, Glenn, Janet F. Bornman, Anthony P. James, and Lucinda J. Black. "A Review of Mushrooms as a Potential Source of Dietary Vitamin D." Nutrients 10, no. 10 (October 2018): 1498. https://doi.org/10.3390/nu10101498.

Chaouali, Nadia, Ines Gana, Amira Dorra, Fathia Khelifi, Anouer Nouioui, Wafa Masri, Ines Belwaer, Hayet Ghorbel, and Abderazzek Hedhili. "Potential Toxic Levels of Cyanide in Almonds (Prunus Amygdalus), Apricot Kernels (Prunus Armeniaca), and Almond Syrup." ISRN Toxicology 2013, (September 2013): 610648. https://doi.org/10.1155/2013/610648.

Committee on Diet and Health Food and Nutrition Board Commission on Life Sciences National Research Council. Diet and Health: Implications for Reducing Chronic Disease Risk. Washington DC: National Academies Press (US), 1989.

"Complementary and Alternative Medicine." St. Luke's Hospital. Accessed February 1, 2021. https://www.stlukes-stl.com/health-content/medicine/33/000238.htm.

Dabrowska, Agata, and Susan Thaul. "How FDA Approves Drugs and Regulates Their Safety and Effectiveness." Congressional Research Service, May 8, 2018. https://fas.org/sgp/crs/misc/R41983.pdf.

"Dietary Supplements." FDA. Last modified August 16, 2019. https://www.fda.gov/food/dietary-supplements.

"Dong Quai." *Medline Plus*. Last modified January 29, 2021. https://medlineplus.gov/druginfo/natural/936.html.

Fernandez-Flores, Angel, Marcela Saeb-Lima, David S Cassarino. "Histopathology of Aging of the Hair Follicle." *Journal of Cutaneous Pathway 46*, no. 7 (July 2019): 508-519. https://doi.org/10.1111/cup.13467.

"Fetal Alcohol Spectrum Disorders (FASDs)." *Centers for Disease Control and Prevention*. Last modified October 8, 2020. https://www.cdc.gov/ncbddd/fasd/alcohol-use.html.

"Folate (Folic Acid) – Vitamin B9." *Harvard Health*. Accessed February 1, 2021. https://www.hsph.harvard.edu/nutritionsource/folic-acid/.

"Folic Acid." *Center for Disease Control and Prevention*. Last modified April 11, 2018. https://www.cdc.gov/ncbddd/folicacid/about.html.

"Folic Acid." *Spina Bifida Association*. Accessed February 1, 2021. https://www.spinabifidaassociation.org/resource/folic-acid/.

Gaziano, John Michael. "Physicians' Health Study II (PHS II)." *NIH: Clinical Trials*. Last modified February 28, 2018. https://clinicaltrials.gov/ct2/show/NCT00270647.

Gernand, Alison D., Kerry J. Schulze, Christine P. Stewart, Keith P. West Jr., and Parul Christian. "Micronutrient Deficiencies in Pregnancy Worldwide: Health Effects and Prevention." *Nature Reviews Endocrinology 12*, no. 5 (June 2016): 274–289. https://doi.org/10.1038/nrendo.2016.37.

Guerrera, Mary P., Stella Lucia Volpe, and Jun James Mao. "Therapeutic Uses of Magnesium." *American Family Physician 80*, no. 2 (July 2009): 157–162. https://www.aafp.org/afp/2009/0715/p157.html#afp20090715p157-b2.

Gutierrez-Mazariegos, Juliana, Maria Theodosiou, Florent Campo-Paysaa, and Michael Schubert. "Vitamin A: A Multifunctional Tool for Development." *Seminars in Cell & Developmental Biology 22*, no. 6 (2011): 603–610. https://doi.org/10.1016/j.semcdb.2011.06.001.

Hansen, Bent-Are, and Oyvind Bruserud. "Hypomagnesemia in Criticall Ill Patients." *Journal of Intensive Care 6*, no. 21 (March 2018). https://doi.org/10.1186/s405060-018-0291-y.

Harwood, John L. "Algae: Critical Sources of Very Long-Chain Polyunsaturated Fatty Acids." *Biomolecules 9*, no. 11 (November 2019): 708. https://doi.org/10.3390/biom9110708.

Healthwise Staff. "Sodium (Na) in Blood." *Michigan Medicine.* Last modified December 8, 2019. https://www.uofmhealth.org/health-library/hw203476.

Herbert, V. "Vitamin B-12: Plant Sources, Requirements, and Assay." *The American Journal of Clinical Nutrition 48*, no. 3 (September 1988): 85--858. https://doi.org/10.1093/ajcn/48.3.852.

Herrmann, W., H. Schorr, K. Purschwitz, F. Rassoul, and V. Richter. "Total Homocysteine, Vitamin B(12), and Total Antioxidant Status in Vegetarians." *Clinical Chemistry 47*, no. 6 (June 2001): 1094-1101. https://pubmed.ncbi.nlm.nih.gov/11375297/.

Holick, Michael F. "Vitamin D Deficiency." *The New Journal of Medicine 357*, no. 3 (2007): 266–281. https://doi.org/10.1056/NEJMra070553.

Hollis, Bruce W., and Carol L. Wagner. "Nutritional Vitamin D Status During Pregnancy: Reasons for Concern." *CMAJ: Canadian Medical Association Journal 174*, no. 9 (April 2006): 1287–90. https://doi.org/10.1503/cmaj.060149.

Hong, Mee Young, Jan Lumibao, Prashila Mistry, Rhonda Saleh, and Eunha Hoh. "Fish Oil Contaminated with Persistent Organic Pollutants Reduces Antioxidant Capacity and Induces Oxidative Stress without Affecting Its Capacity to Lower Lipid Concentrations and Systemic Inflammation in Rats." *The Journal of Nutrition 145*, no. 5 (May 2015): 939–44. https://doi.org/10.3945/jn.114.206607.

Hossein-Nezhad, Arash, and Michael F. Holick. "Vitamin D for Health: A Global Perspective." *Mayo Clinic Proceedings 88*, no. 7 (June 2013): 720–755. https://doi.org/10.1016/j.mayocp.2013.05.011.

Institute of Medicine. *Dietary Reference Intakes for Calcium and Vitamin D*. Washington DC: National Academy Press, 2011.

Jeong, Harin, Sunjin Hong, Yunjeong Heo, Hosun Chun, Daeseong Kim, Jongtae Park, and Mo-yeol Kang. "Vitamin D Status and Associated Occupational Factors in Korean Wage Workers: Data from the 5th Korea National Health and Nutrition Examination Survey (KNHANES 2010-2012)." *Annals of Occupational and Environmental Medicine 26*, no. 28 (September 2014). https://doi.org/10.1186/s40557-014-0028-x.

Klein, Eric A., Ian M. Thompson Jr., Catherine M. Tangen, John J. Crowley, M. Scott Lucia, Phyllis J. Goodman, Lori M. Minasian, Leslie G. Ford, Howard L. Parnes, J. Michael Gaziano, Daniel D. Karp, Michael M. Lieber, Philip J. Walther, Laurence Klotz, J. Kellogg Parsons, Joseph L. Chin, Amy K. Darke, Scott M. Lippman, Gary E. Goodman, Frank L. Meyskens Jr., and Laurence H. Baker. "Vitamin E and the Risk of Prostate Cancer: The Selenium and Vitamin E Cancer Prevention Trial (SELECT)." *JAMA 306*, no. 14 (October 2011): 1549–1556. https://doi.org/10.1001/jama.2011.1437.

Krause, Lydia, Erica Cirino, and Ana Gotter. "Pernicious Anemia," *Healthline*, May 13, 2020. https://www.healthline.com/health/pernicious-anemia.

Licea, Melkorka. "Woman Says She Suffered Liver Failure after Taking 'Health Supplement." *NY Post*, January 3, 2020. https://nypost.com/2020/01/03/woman-says-she-suffered-liver-failure-after-taking-health-supplement//.

Ma, Yuan, Feng J. He, and Graham A. MacGregor. "High Salt Intake: Independent Risk Factor for Obesity." *Hypertension 66*, no. 4 (October 2015): 843–849. https://doi.org/10.1161/HYPERTENSIONAHA.115.05948.

Madell, Robin. "What Is Phosphorus and Why Is It Important?." *Healthline*. Last modified July 31, 2020. https://www.healthline.com/health/phosphorus-in-diet.

"Magnesium." *NIH: Office of Dietary Supplements*. Last modified March 24, 2020. https://ods.od.nih.gov/factsheets/Magnesium-Consumer/.

"Magnesium Rich Food." *Cleveland Clinic*. Last modified November 24, 2020. https://my.clevelandclinic.org/health/articles/15650-magnesium-rich-food.

Maia, Sabina Bastos, Alex Sandro Rolland Souza, Maria de Fátima Costa Caminha, Suzana Lins de Silva, Rachel de Sá Barreto Luna Callou Cruz, Camila Carvalho dos Santos, and Malaquias Batista Filho. "Vitamin A and Pregnancy: A Narrative Review." *Nutrients* 11, no. 3 (March 2019): 681. https://doi.org/10.3390/nu11030681.

Maranduca, Minela Aida, Daciana Branisteanu, Dragomir Nicolae Serban, Daniel Constantin Branisteanu, Gabriela Stoleriu, Nicuta Manolache, and Lonela Lacramioara Serban. "Synthesis and Physiological Implication of Melanic Pigments." *Oncology Letters* 17, no. 5 (February 2019): 4183–4187. https://doi.org/10.3892/ol.2019.10071.

May, Sandra. "Minerals (Lesson 8)." *LSU Agriculture Center*, February 25, 2019. https://www.lsuagcenter.com/topics/food_health/education_resources/eatsmart/lessons/minerals-lesson-8.

Mayo Clinic Staff. "Omega-3 in Fish: How Eating Fish Helps Your Heart." *Mayo Clinic*, September 28, 2019. https://www.mayoclinic.org/diseases-conditions/heart-disease/in-depth/omega-3/art-20045614.

Mayo Clinic Staff. "Preeclampsia." *Mayo Clinic*, March 19, 2020. https://www.mayoclinic.org/diseases-conditions/preeclampsia/symptoms-causes/syc-20355745.

Mayo Clinic Staff. "Prenatal Vitamins: Why They Matter, How to Choose." *Mayo Clinic*, May 1, 2020. https://www.mayoclinic.org/healthy-lifestyle/pregnancy-week-by-week/in-depth/prenatal-vitamins/art-20046945.

Mayo Clinic Staff. "Rickets." *Mayo Clinic*, May 14, 2019. https://www.mayoclinic.org/diseases-conditions/rickets/symptoms-causes/syc-20351943.

Mayo Clinic Staff. "Vitamin E." *Mayo Clinic*, November 13, 2020. https://www.mayoclinic.org/drugs-supplements-vitamin-e/art-20364144.

"Minerals." *Medline Plus*. Last modified October 19, 2020. https://medlineplus.gov/minerals.html.

Nair, Rathish, and Arun Maseeh. "Vitamin D: The "Sunshine" Vitamin." *Journal of Pharmacology & Pharmacotherapeutics* 3, no. 2 (April-June 2012): 118–126. https://doi.rg/10.4103/0976-500X.95506.

National Institutes of Health. *Dietary Reference Intakes for Calcium, Phosphorus, Magnesium, Vitamin D, and Fluoride.* Washington DC: National Academies Press, 1997.

National Research Council (US). *Copper in Drinking Water.* Washington DC: National Academies Press (US), 2000.

Navarro, Victor, Ikhlas Khan, Einar Björnsson, Leonard B. Seeff, Jose Serrano, and Jay H. Hoofnagle. "Liver Injury from Herbal and Dietary Supplements." *Hepatology 65*, no. 1 (July 2017): 363-373. https://doi.org/10.1002/hep.28813.

"Nutrition During Pregnancy." *The American College of Obstetricians and Gynecologists*, June 2020. https://www.acog.org/womens-health/faqs/nutrition-during-pregnancy.

Oh, Christina, Emily C. Keats, and Zulfiqar A. Bhutta. "Vitamin and Mineral Supplementation During Pregnancy and Maternal, Birth, Child Health and Development Outcomes in Low- and Middle- Income Countries: A Systematic Review and Meta-Analysis." *Nutrients 12*, no. 2 (2012): 491. https://doi.org/10.3390/nu12020491.

"Omega-3 Fatty Acids." *NIH: Office of Dietary Supplements*. Last modified October 1, 2020. https://ods.od.nih.gov/factsheets/Omega3FattyAcids-HealthProfessional/.

Pandit, A. N., and S. A. Bhave. "Copper and Indian Childhood Cirrhosis." *Indian Pediatrics 20*, no. 12 (December 1983): 893-899. https://pubmed.ncbi.nlm.nih.gov/6676301/.

"Phosphorus in Diet." *Medline Plus*. Last modified January 5, 2021. https://medlineplus.gov/ency/article/002424.htm.

Plant Based News. "Which Supplements Are Necessary? Doctors Weigh In." March 26, 2020, video, 5:19. https://www.youtube.com/watch?v=xwcJI5d5G9k.

Ryan, Alan S., Michelle A. Keske, James P. Hoffman, and Edward B. Nelson. "Clinical Overview of Algal-Docosahexaenoic Acid: Effects on Triglyceride Levels and Other Cardiovascular Risk Factors." *American Journal of Therapeutics 16*, no. 2 (March-April 2009): 183–192. https://doi.org/10.1097/MJT.0b013e31817fe2be.

"Salt and Sodium." *Harvard Health*. Accessed February 13, 2021. https://www.hsph.harvard.edu/nutritionsource/salt-and-sodium/.

"Salt: The Role of Potassium and Sodium in Your Diet." *Centers for Disease Control and Prevention*. Last modified June 29, 2018. https://www.cdc.gov/salt/potassium.htm.

Scialli, Anthony R. "Does Vitamin A Cause Birth Defects?." *Relias Media*, November 1, 2001. https://www.reliasmedia.com/articles/74324-does-vitamin-a-cause-birth-defects.

Sesso, Howard D., Julie E. Buring, William G. Christen, Tobias Kurth, Charlene Belanger, Jean MacFadyem, Vadim Bubes, JoAnn E. Manson, Robert J. Glynn, and J. Michael Gaziano. "Vitamins E and C in the Prevention of Cardiovascular Disease in Men: The Physicians' Health Study II Randomized Controlled Trial." *JAMA 300*, no. 18 (November 2008): 2123–33. https://doi/org/10.1001/jama.2008.600.

"Should You Consider Taking a Fish Oil Supplements?." *Harvard Health*, December 2017. https://www.hcalth.harvard.edu/heart-health/should-you-consider-taking-a-fish-oil-supplement.

Silva, Mariana Costa, and Tania Weber Furlanetto. "Intestinal Absorption of Vitamin D: A Systematic Review." *Nutrition Reviews 76*, no. 1 (2018): 60–76. https://doi.org/10.1093/nutrit/nux034.

Siscovick, David S., Thomas A.. Barringer, Amanda M. Fretts, Jason H. Y. Wu, AAlice H. Lichtenstein, Rebecca B. Costello, Penny M. Kris-Etherton, Terry A. Jacobson, Mary B. Engler,

Heather M. Aalger, Lawrence J. Appel, and Dariush Mozaffarian. "Omega-3 Polyunsaturated Fatty Acid (Fish Oil) Supplementation and the Prevention of Clinical Cardiovascular Disease." *AHA Journal 135*, (April 2017): e867–e884. https://doi.org/10.1161/CIR.0000000000000482.

Soma-Pillay, Priya, Nelson-Piercy Catherine, Heli Tolppanean, and Alexandre Mebazaa. "Physiological Changes in Pregnancy." *Cardiovascular Journal of Africa 27*, no. 2 (March-April 2016); 80–91 https://doi.org/10.5830/CVJA-2016-021.

Spence, John David. "B Vitamin Therapy for Homocysteine: Renal Function and Vitamin B12 Determine Cardiovascular Outcomes." *Clinical Chemistry and Laboratory Medicine 51*, no. 3 (March 2013): 633-637. https://doi.org/10.1515/cclm-2012-0465.

Starace, Michela, Aurora Alessandrini, Nicolo Brandi, and Bianca Maria Piraccini. "Use of Nail Dermoscopy in the Management of Melanonychia: Review." *Dermatology Practical & Conceptual 9*, no. 1 (January 2019): 38–43. https://doi.org/10.5826/dpc.0901a10.

"Step 2 in MTHFR Support: How to Choose the Right B12 for You." *MTHRF Support Australia.* Accessed February 1, 2021. https://mthfrsupport.com.au/2016/09/step-2-in-mthfr-support-how-to-choose-the-right-b12-for-you/.

"Supplements: A Scorecard." *Harvard Health*, April 2012. https://www.health.harvard.edu/staying-healthy/supplements-a-scorecard.

Tanna, Bhakti, and Avinash Mishra. "Metabolites Unravel Nutra-ceutical Potential of Edible Seaweeds: An Emerging Source of Functional Food." *Comprehensive Reviews in Food Science and Food Safety 17*, no. 6 (October 2018). https://doi.org/10.1111/1541-4337.12396.

Ted Talk. Neal Barnard: Power Foods for the Brain." September 20, 2016, video, 17:00. https://www.youtube.com/watch?v=v_ONFix_e4k.

Tello, Monique. "Vitamin D: What's the "Right" Level?." *Harvard Health*. Last modified April 16, 2020. https://www.health.harvard.edu/blog/vitamin-d-whats-right-level-2016121910893.

Tello, Monique. "What Patients- and Doctors- Need to Know About Vitamins and Supplements." *Harvard Health*, March 16, 2018. https://www.health.harvard.edu/blog/patients-doctors-know-vitamins-supplements-2018031613418.

The Doctors. "Woman Almost Dies After Taking Daily Supplements?." February 19, 2020, video, 4:50. https://www.youtube.com/watch?v=zyxYSqvMZIM.

Tripkovic, Laura, Helen Lambert, Kathryn Hart, Colin P. Smith, Giselda Bucca, Simon Penson, Gemma Chope, Elina Hyppönen, Jacqueline Berry, Reinhold Vieth, and Susan Lanham-New. "Comparison of Vitamin D2 and Vitamin D3 Supplementation in Raising Serum 25-Hydroxyvitamin D Status: A Systematic Review and Meta-Analysis." *The American Journal of Clinical Nutrition 95*, no. 6 (May 2012): 1357-1364. https://doi.org/10.3945/ajcn.111.031070.

Tripkovic, Laura, Louise R. Wilson, Kathryn Hart, Sig Johnsen, Simon de Lusignan, Colin P. Smith, Giselda Bucca, Simon Penson, Gemme Chope, Ruan Elliot, Elina Hyppönen, Jacqueline L. Berry, and Susan A. Lanham-New. "Daily Supplementation with 15 μG Vitamin D2 Compared with Vitamin D3 to Increase Wintertime 25-Hydroxyvitamin D Status in Healthy South Asian and White European Women: A 12-Wk Randomized, Placebo-Controlled Food-Fortification Trial." *The American Journal of Clinical Nutrition 106*, no. 2 (2017): 481–490. https://doi.org/10.3945/ajcn.116.138693.

Van de Lagemaat, Erik E., Lisette C.P.G.M de Groot, and Ellen G.H.M Van den Heuvel. "Vitamin B12 in Relation to Oxidative Stress: A Systematic Review." Nutrients 11, no. 2 (February 2019): 482. https://doi.org/10.3390/nu11020482.

"Vitamin B12." *NIH: Office of Dietary Supplements.* Last modified January 15, 2021. https://ods.od.nih.gov/factsheets/VitaminB12-Consumer/.

"Vitamin D." *NIH: Office of Dietary Supplements.* Last modified on October 9, 2020. https://ods.od.nih.gov/factsheets/Vitamind-HealthProfessional/.

"Vitamin D and Your Health: Breaking Old Rules, Raising New Hopes." *Harvard Health.* Last modified May 17, 2019. https://www.health.harvard.edu/staying-healthy/vitamin-d-and-your-health-breaking-old-rules-raising-new-hopes.

"Vitamin D for Milk and Milk Alternatives." *FDA*, January 4, 2018. https://www.fda.gov/food/food-additives-petitions/vitamin-d-milk-and-milk-alternatives.

"Vitamin E." *NIH: Office of Dietary Supplements.* Last modified July 31, 2020. https://ods.od.nih.gov/factsheets/VitaminE-Health-Professional/.

"Vitamin K." *NIH: Office of Dietary Supplements.* Last modified February 24, 2020. https://ods.od.nih.gov/factsheets/VitaminK-Consume.

"Vitamins and Minerals." *Harvard Health: HelpGuide.* Accessed February 1, 2021. https://www.helpguide.org/harvard/vitamins-and-minerals.htm.

Vogtman, Holly. "Dietary Supplement Use Reaches All Time High." *CRN USA,* September 30, 2019. https://www.crnusa.org/newsroom/dietary-supplement-use-reaches-all-time-high.

Weil, Andrew. "PCBs in Fish Oil Supplements." *Dr Weil,* July 8, 2010. https://www.drweil.com/vitamins-supplements-herbs/supplements-remedies/pcbs-in-fish-oil-supplements/.

Westphalen, Dena. "Supplements During Pregnancy: What's Safe and What's Not." *Healthline.* Last modified August 13, 2020. https://www.healthline.com/nutrition/supplements-during-pregnancy#supplements-to-avoid.

"What You Need to Know about Dietary Supplements." *FDA.* Last modified November 29, 2017. https://www.fda.gov/food/buy-store-serve-safe-food/what-you-need-know-about-dietary-supplements.

BREAKFAST

Affinitia, Antonio, Loredana Catalani, Giovanna Cecchetto, Gianfranco De Lorenzo, Dario Dililo, Giorgio Donegani, Lucia Fransos, Fabio Lucidi, Chiara Mameli, Elisa Manna, Paolo Marconi, Giuseppe Mele, Laura Minestroni, Massimo Montanari, Mario Morcellini, Giuseppe Rovera, Giuseppe Rotilio, Marco Sachet, and Gian Vincenzo Zuccotti. "Breakfast: A Multidisciplinary Approach." *Italian Journal of Pediatrics 39*, no. 44 (July 2013). https://doi.org/10.1186/1824-7288-39-44.

Betts, James A., Judith D. Richardson, Enhad A. Chowdhury, Geoffrey D. Holman, Kostas Tsintzas, and Dylan Thompson. "The Causal Role of Breakfast in Energy Balance and Health: A Randomized Controlled Trial in Lean Adults." *The American Journal of Clinical Nutrition 100*, no. 2 (August 2014): 539-547. https://doi.org/10.3945/ajcn.114.083402.

Cabo, Rafael de, and Mark P. Mattson. "Effects of Intermittent Fasting on Health, Aging, and Disease." *The New England Journal of Medicine 381*, no. 26 (December 2019): 2541–2551. https://doi.org/10.1056/NEJMra1905136.

Fan, Shelly. "The Fat-Fueled Brain: Unnatural or Advantageous?." *Scientific American* (blog), October 1, 2013. https://blogs.scientificamerican.com/mind-guest-blog/the-fat-fueled-brain-unnatural-or-advantageous/.

"Grape-Nuts." *Mr. Breakfast.* Accessed January 30, 2021. https://www.mrbreakfast.com/cereal_detail.asp?id=175.

Horne, Jeffrey L. Anderson, John F. Carlquist, Brent Muhlestein, Donald L. Lappé, Heidi T. May, Boudi Kfoury, Oxana Galenko,

Amy R. Butler, Dylan P. Nelson, Kimberly D. Brusisholz, Tami L. Bair, and Samin Panahi. "Study Finds Routine Periodic Fasting is Good for Your Health, and Your Heart." *Intermountain Medical Center*, April 3, 2011. https://www.eurekalert.org/pub_releases/2011-04/imc-sfr033111.php.

Lennon, Troy. "How the Kellogg Brothers Influenced the way Westerners Eat Breakfast." *Daily Telegraph*, August 8, 2018. https://www.dailytelegraph.com.au/news/how-the-kellogg-brothers-influenced-the-way-westerners-eat-breakfast/news-story/7478e97f93d98c466454ac970a88e9ad.

Longo, Valter D., and Satchidananda Panda. "Fasting, Circadian Rhythms, and Time Restricted Feeding in Healthy Lifespan." *Cell Metabolism* 23, no. 6 (2016): 1048–1059. https://doi.org/10.1016/j.cmet.2016.06.001.

"Oldest Cereals Ever Created." *Oldest*. Accessed January 30, 2021. https://www.oldest.org/food/cereals/.

Pruitt, Sarah. "How an Accidental Invention Changed What Americans Eat for Breakfast?." *History*. Last modified August 5, 2019. https://www.history.com/news/cereal-breakfast-origins-kellogg.

"Satchidananda Panda." *Salk Edu*. Accessed January 30, 2021. https://www.salk.edu/scientist/satchidananda-panda/.

Shaw, P., J. Walton, and P. Jakeman. "The Effects of the Special K Challenge on Body Composition and Biomarkers of Metabolic Health in Healthy Adults." *Journal of Nutrition and Health*

Sciences 2, no. 4 (November 2015). https://doi.org 10.15744/2393-9060.2.403.

"Skipping Breakfast May Increase Coronary Heart Disease Risk." *Harvard Health*, July 23, 2013. https://www.hsph.harvard.edu/news/features/skipping-breakfast-may-increase-coronary-heart-disease-risk/.

Stephen, Gin. *Fast. Feast. Repeat.* New York: St. Martin's Press, 2020.

Tello, Monique. "Intermittent Fasting: Surprising Update." *Harvard Health*, June 29, 2018. https://www.health.harvard.edu/blog/intermittent-fasting-surprising-update-2018062914156.

"Why You Should Eat Breakfast." *Rush Edu*. Accessed January 30, 2021. https://www.rush.edu/news/why-you-should-eat-breakfast.

Zelman, Kathleen M. "The Special K Challenge." *WebMD*. Accessed January 30, 2021. https://www.webmd.com/diet/features/the-special-k-challenge#1.

DESSERT

Allison, Kelly C., and Ellen Tarves. "Treatment of Night Eating Syndrome." *The Psychiatric Clinic of North America 34*, no.4 (September 2011): 785–96. Https://doi.org/10.1016/j.psc.2011.08.002.

Barnes, Christopher M. "Will Blue Light Glasses Improve Your Sleep?." Harvard Business Review, October 14, 2020. https://hbr.org/2020/10/will-blue-light-glasses-improve-your-sleep.

Bowen, Richard. "Gastrointestinal Transit: How Long Does It Take?." *VIVO Pathophysiology*. Accessed February 14, 2021. http://www.vivo.colostate.edu/hbooks/pathphys/digestion/basics/transit.html.

Bowen, Richard. "The Pineal Gland and Melatonin." *VIVO Pathophysiology*. Last modified November 2018. http://www.vivo.colostate.edu/hbooks/pathphys/endocrine/otherendo/pineal.html.

Breus, Michael J. "Magnesium – How it Affects Your Sleep." *Psychology Today (blog)*, May 2, 2018. https://www.psychologytoday.com/us/blog/sleep-newzzz/201805/magnesium-how-it-affects-your-sleep.

Healthwise Staff. "Night Eating Syndrome." *Michigan Medicine*, May 28, 2019. https://www.uofmhealth.org/health-library/aa107116.

"Heartburn Keeping You Up at Night?." *GI Society: Canadian Society of Intestinal Research*. Accessed February 15, 2021. https://badgut.org/information-centre/a-z-digestive-topics/heartburn-keeping-night/.

Hines, Jennifer. "Food for Sleep: The Best and Worst Foods for Getting Sleep." *Alaska Sleep Education Center*, June 24, 2019. https://www.alaskasleep.com/blog/foods-for-sleep-list-best-worst-foods-getting-sleep-0.

Inam, Qurrat-ul-Aen, Huma Ikram, Erum Shireen, and Darakhshan Jabeen Haleem. "Effects of Sugar Rich Diet on the Brain Serotonin, Hyperphagia and Anxiety in Animal Model of Both Genders." *Pakistan Journal of Pharmaceutical Sciences 29*, no. 3 (2016): 757-763. https://pubmed.ncbi.nlm.nih.gov/27166525/.

Krueger, James M. "The Role of Cytokines in Sleep Regulation." *Current Pharamaceutical Design 14*, no.32 (2008): 3408–16. https://doi.org/10.2174/138161208786549281.

"Magnesium Rich Food." *Cleveland Clinic.* Last modified November 24, 2020. https://my.clevelandclinic.org/health/articles/15650-magnesium-rich-food.

Mayo Clinic Staff. "Insomnia." *Mayo Clinic*, October 15, 2016. https://www.mayoclinic.org/diseases-conditions/insomnia/symptoms-causes/syc-20355167.

"Melatonin: What You Need to Know." *NIH.* Last modified October 2019. https://www.nccih.nih.gov/health/melatonin-what-you-need-to-know.

National Sleep Foundation. "How Much Caffeine Should You Really Be Having?." *Sleep.org.* Accessed on February 15, 2021. https://www.sleep.org/how-much-caffiene-should-i-have/.

Nehlig, Astrid. "The Neuroprotective Effects of Cocoa Flavanol and its Influence on Cognitive Performance." *British Journal of Clinical Pharmacology 75*, no. 3 (March 2013): 716–27. https://doi.org/10.1111/j.1365-2125.2012.04378.x.

Pace-Schott, Edward F. "Serotonin and Dreaming." *Serotonin and Sleep: Molecular, Functional and Clinical Aspects* (2008): 307-324. https://doi.org/10.1007/978-3-7643-8561-3_12.

"REM Sleep and Our Dreaming Lives." *S+ ResMed*. Accessed February 15, 2021. http://sleep.mysplus.com/library/category3/ REM_Sleep_and_Our_Dreaming_Lives.html.

Singh, Abhinav. "Alcohol and Sleep." *Sleep Foundation*. Last modified September 4, 2020. https://www.sleepfoundation.org/ nutrition/alcohol-and-sleep.

Sissons, Claire. "How to Boost Serotonin and Improve Mood." *Medical News Today*, July 10, 2018. https://www.medical-newstoday.com/articles/322416#eight-foods-that-naturally-boost-serotonin.

St-Onge, Marie-Pierre, Amy Roberts, Ari Schechter, and Adrindam Roy Choudhury. "Fiber and Saturated Fat are Associated with Sleep Arousals and Slow Wave Sleep." *Journal of Clinical Sleep Medicine 12*, no. 1 (January 2016): 19–24. https://doi.org/10.5664/jcsm.5384.

Stein, Michael D., and Peter D. Friedmann. "Disturbed Sleep and Its Relationship to Alcohol Use." *Substance Abuse 26*, no. 1 (March 2005): 1–13. https://doi.org/10.1300/j465v25n01_01.

Taheri, Shahrad, Ling Lin, Diane Austin, Terry Young, and Emmanuel Mignot. "Short Sleep Duration is Associated with Reduced Leptin, Elevated Ghrelin, and Increased Body Mass Index." *PLoS Medicine 1*, no.3 (December 2004): e62. https://doi.org/10.1371/journal.pmed.0010062.

Tosini, Gianluca, Ian Ferguson, and Kazuo Tsubota. "Effects of Blue Light on the Circadian System and Eye Physiology."

Molecular Vision 22 (January 2016): 61–72. https://www.ncbi.
nlm.nih.gov/pmc/articles/PMC4734149/.

University of Bristol. "Chocolate Is the Most Widely Craved Food,
but Is It Really Addictive?." *ScienceDaily*, September 12, 2007.
https://www.sciencedaily.com/releases/2007/09/070911073921.
htm.

Ursin, Reidun. "Serotonin and Sleep." *Sleep Medicine Reviews 6*, no.
1 (2002): 55–69. https://doi.org/10.1053/smrv.2001.0174.

Vandergriendt, Carly. "What's the Difference Between Dopamine and Serotonin?." *Healthline*. Last modified July 16, 2020.
https://www.healthline.com/health/dopamine-vs-serotonin.

Volkow, Nora D., Dardo Tomasi, Gene-Jack Wang, Frank Telang,
Joanna S. Fowler, Jean Logan, Helene Benveniste, Ron Kim,
Panayotis K. Thanos, and Sergi Ferré. "Evidence That Sleep
Deprivation Downregulates Dopamine d2r in Ventral Stri-
atum in the Human Brain." *The Journal of Neuroscience 32*,
no. 19 (May 2012): 6711–6717. https://doi.org/10.1523/JNEURO-
SCI.0045-12.2012.

"What Is Night Eating Syndrome?." *WebMD*. Accessed on February
15, 2021. https://www.webmd.com/mental-health/eating-disor-
ders/binge-eating-disorder/what-is-night-eating-syndrome.

Yannielli, Paola C., Penny C. Molyneuz, Mary E. Harrington, and
Diego A. Golombek. "Ghrelin Effects on the Circadian System
of Mice." *The Journal of Neuroscience: The Office Journal of the
Society for Neuroscience 27*, no. 11 (March 2007): 2890–2895.
https://doi.org/10.1523/JNEUROSCI.3913-06.2007.

Lightning Source UK Ltd.
Milton Keynes UK
UKHW022310060223
416578UK00007B/909/J